The Miracle Ball Method
for Pregnancy

The Miracle
for

Relieve Back Pain, Ease Labor, Reduce Stress,
Regain a Flat Belly, and More

Ball Method
Pregnancy

by **Elaine Petrone**

Workman Publishing • *New York*

Copyright © 2011 by Elaine Petrone

Design copyright © by Workman Publishing

Photographs copyright © by Evan Sklar
Illustrations copyright © by Nicole Kaufman

Library of Congress Cataloging-in-Publication Data is available.

ISBN 978-0-7611-6097-7

Workman books are available at special discounts when purchased in bulk for premiums
and sales promotions as well as for fund-raising or educational use. Special editions or
book excerpts also can be created to specification. For details, contact the Special Sales
Director at the address below or send an e-mail to specialmarkets@workman.com.

Workman Publishing Company, Inc.
225 Varick Street
New York, NY 10014-4381
www.workman.com

Printed in China
First printing March 2011
10 9 8 7 6 5 4 3 2 1

Note to Readers

This book is not intended as a substitute for medical advice. Therefore before trying any of the exercises described in this book, you should consult your obstetrician/gynecologist or other health care provider. Neither the author nor the publisher shall be liable or responsible for any loss or damage allegedly arising from your performing any of the exercises in this book.

Dedication

*Women usually take care of everyone else
before they take care of themselves. My mother
once told me that she waited for her family's
problems to be solved before she could start living
her life. That never happened. So, do something
good for yourself. Don't wait. Start now.*

*This book is dedicated to my mom and
to all the women past, present, and future
who have gone on this journey with me.*

Contents

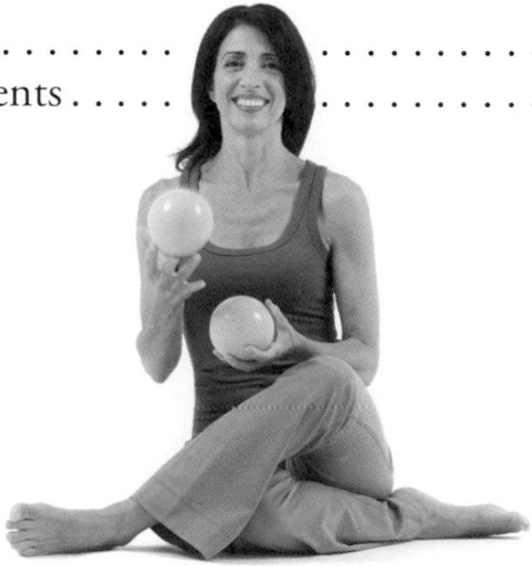

Foreword

The majority of women will experience discomfort during the course of pregnancy. Elaine Petrone's method offers a non-invasive, low impact, and financially practical solution to ease the tensions associated with pregnancy and help women find relief.

In this book, Elaine takes her proven techniques for realigning the body with muscle relaxation and proper breathing, and adapts them for pregnancy. The passive realignment process is ideally suited for the pregnant woman who may find strenuous exercise difficult. By simply using their weight to realign and adjust their bodies, women can better accommodate the major physiological changes they experience during pregnancy. In addition, the focus on proper breathing is essential in preparing for a successful delivery.

Elaine walks the reader through the fundamental "Ball" concepts and then provides step-by-step directions that make these simple moves and positions easy to master. The low-impact *Miracle Ball Method for Pregnancy* is a tool that most pregnant woman will find useful at any stage in their pregnancy and the months that follow.

Lance R. Bruck, M.D.
CHAIRMAN, DEPARTMENT OF OBSTETRICS
AND GYNECOLOGY, STAMFORD HOSPITAL
STAMFORD, CONNECTICUT

Introduction

The idea for this book grew out of my own prenatal and postpartum experience as well as the experiences of thousands of women who have attended my classes over the years. So many suffered from pregnancy-related issues such as sciatic pain, backaches, weight problems, elevated stress levels, TMJ, and more. They would tell me: "I've had sciatic pain ever since having my third child," or "I can't get my shape back." One mother of twins told me she had chronic stomach discomfort since giving birth—25 years ago! After practicing the Miracle

Ball Method, they found that their pain was relieved. Their muscles adjusted, allowing the shape of their body to improve. They lost inches. They stood taller. They were more relaxed.

Pregnancy can be a wonderful time. It can also be a time of physical discomfort and emotional stress. Over nine months, your body changes dramatically, literally reshaping itself in order to house and nourish your baby. As your belly grows, you may experience backaches, indigestion, and difficulty breathing, sleeping, and moving. Compounded with the practical and emotional concerns that go along with preparing for a new child, it's no wonder that many pregnant women feel overwhelmed.

The solution for most of these pregnancy-related complaints—both physical *and* emotional—is the same: Reduce your muscle tension. *The Miracle Ball Method for Pregnancy* teaches you to let go of tension, making your muscles supple enough to allow your body to realign and reshape. Simply by resting on the balls and focusing on your breath, you can relieve aches and pains, lower your stress levels, and focus your energy on enjoying your pregnancy and the following months with your new baby.

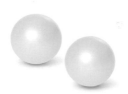

My Story

I developed the Miracle Ball Method out of my own experience with chronic back pain. I tried various therapies and found little relief. One day, I rested my knee on a ball and simply let its weight give in to gravity. The tension released and my pain dramatically lessened. I listened to my body and continued to experiment with resting different body parts on the ball. I began to make the connection that if I worked less, I got better results. Within months I went from walking with a limp to being in the best shape of my life.

That's why, when I became pregnant with twins, I was sure I would sail through the nine months. Instead, I noticed that my posture was rounding, and my breathing was labored. My belly was growing so large that even walking was a challenge! Then I realized that relief was at my fingertips. I tailored my method to target the areas that were plaguing me and the results were amazing.

My postpartum period presented an entirely new set of challenges. Carrying such large babies (7 pounds each!) had left my body a mess. I had what is called "twin skin," excess skin that I could roll up and tuck into my pants. On top of that, my stress levels soared. The method was more essential than ever.

Gradually my muscles began to lengthen and my body to realign. I began to regain my shape as well as my confidence and energy, allowing me to do the real work of taking care of my babies.

Moms and the Miracle Ball

Millions of people found relief from my previous books, *The Miracle Ball Method,* published in 2003, and *The Portable Miracle Ball Method,* published in 2006. I've received letters from readers all over the globe saying that they were finally free from issues like back pain, sciatic pain, sleeplessness, headaches, and more, thanks to this program. Many of them, like the women in my classes, were pregnant or dealing with issues related to their pregnancies. This book is for them.

We women, especially moms, try so hard to get everything done, we leave little time for ourselves. We may not have the spare hours or funds for a gym or a personal trainer but healing our body of its aches and pains and regaining our shape shouldn't be a luxury. This method is ideal for the overworked, stressed mom or mom-to-be because it doesn't require you to do much more than rest on the ball and breathe. One ball placement, if done well, will create a chain reaction throughout your whole body. Simply by feeling the weight and releasing your tension, your body can recover from the miraculous work of carrying and delivering your baby. So don't wait. Start now.

CHAPTER ONE

The Miracle Ball Method and Pregnancy

The Miracle Ball Method is deceptively simple: You place the ball under whichever body part you've chosen, take note of your breath, and let your weight be absorbed by the ball. As you slowly release your excess tension, over time your muscles will become supple enough to allow your bones to realign and your posture to improve.

Your body has a natural recovery and realignment system—restoring its balance can prevent common pregnancy complaints like sciatic pain, neck and shoulder strain, and discomfort in feet and knees. It will also improve your shape. Think of it this way: Your muscles are like the clothing you put over your skeleton. If you wore a piece of clothing that felt uncomfortable, you would tailor it until it fit correctly. When your muscles don't feel like they "fit" right, it's because the tension is holding them in an uncomfortable spot. The aches and pains felt during pregnancy are often the result of your body fighting the natural postural adjustments your body makes to accommodate the baby growing inside of you. These physical adjustments are necessary to support your expanding belly, and are out of your control. However, you *can* control the muscle tension.

Breaking the Cycle

Excess muscle tension can come from three sources: the lingering effects of an accident or injury; emotional or life stress; and alignment issues such as poor posture. Just one of these pre-existing conditions can make it harder for your body to adjust during pregnancy. Many of us have all three.

When you feel stress or experience negative changes in your body's alignment, your muscles tighten, and when your muscles tighten they resist change and cause you to take shallower breaths. When your breathing becomes shallow, you take in even less oxygen, which causes your muscles to tighten even more. The tighter your muscles become, and the less oxygen you take in, the harder it is for your body to recover. As a result, stress and tension continue to build in those muscles, often spreading throughout your body. It becomes a vicious cycle.

Imagine holding a tennis ball as tightly as you possibly can for hours without letting go— or even days. Can you imagine how awful the

Cycle of Pain

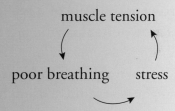

muscle tension

poor breathing   stress

pain would be? But even if you did finally relax
your hand, what would happen? It would remain
curved in a claw shape and probably take hours
to relax into its normal state. We hold so much
tension in our bodies that, despite intense pain,
we are unable to relax our muscles simply because

our bodies have forgotten how. We get into what are called "habits of movement." As with any bad habit, we may not be aware of it while we are doing it, but we often pay the price afterward.

The cycle of pain is difficult to break unless you can find a way to relieve the tension in your overworked muscles. But how do you reduce muscle tension? By using what I call your body formula:

Your Body Formula
Weight + Breathing = Release of Tension

The first essential piece of the formula is "weight." You will notice this word throughout the book, so I want to clarify that I am referring not to the numbers on a scale, but rather to a feeling or an awareness of your body. As you move, your body understands how much effort to use based on an innate sense of the weight of its different parts and how they relate to one another. By using your body formula—combining the weight of the body part you are working with the pull of gravity and your breathing—you will begin to notice how you are holding your muscles and preventing them from resting. By breathing and feeling your weight on the balls, you will learn how to let go and allow your body to adjust naturally.

How Pregnancy Changes Your Body

The body is remarkable and is perfectly able to adapt to the physical changes of pregnancy. But because most of us start pregnancy with excess muscle tension and alignment issues, we find ourselves plagued with discomfort. At the root of these changes is the pelvis (illustrated below). *Pelvis* is the Greek word for "bowl." The pelvic cavity is where you carry your baby. It is also the hub of your skeleton (I call it the "great connector")—your lower back connects to the top of your pelvis, and your legs connect to the bottom, close to your sitz bones (the two points at the base of the pelvis). Think of it as a hinge. During pregnancy, your pelvic bowl "spills" or tilts forward as the baby gets bigger, rotating your hips and causing a chain reaction throughout your whole body, potentially leading to backaches, sciatic pain, and that stomach pouch that never seems to go away.

In addition, as the uterus grows, the baby pushes up under the rib cage, which can put pressure on the diaphragm (the muscle that sits flat across your torso just below your lungs).

This can make breathing difficult. Without the benefit of good breathing, your muscles don't receive the oxygen they need, so they become even tighter, causing more stress and further postural misalignment.

Like children's building blocks, your head, rib cage, and pelvis balance in relation to one another. When one part is tight or out of alignment, your whole body is affected. By using the balls and improving your breathing, the tight muscles will ease and the tilting of the pelvis will lessen, allowing the lower back and neck to lengthen, the muscles around the rib cage to expand, and the shoulders to relax.

You should never feel like you are holding your pelvis, rib cage, and head stiffly in place in order to reach perfect alignment or posture. Unlike actual building blocks, your body parts are made to move. They will never remain stacked one on top of the other in a static position. You need to allow your body to move naturally and adjust to find balance. That is true strength.

Your Body Dialogue

An essential component to the Miracle Ball Method is learning how to read your body's signals. Often when we are in pain or feeling stressed or preoccupied, we don't listen to our bodies—this is especially true during pregnancy. The only time we stop and feel is when we're getting a pain signal. Pain is your body's way of telling you that you need to make an adjustment. But often, by the time you've hit the point of pain, it's too late for your body to be able to self-adjust.

When you feel frozen with tension, it's common to try to force your body into what you think the correct position might be. But thinking

Check In with Your Body Dialogue

1. Note how your body feels.
2. Choose what you're going to do about it.
3. Note your body's responses.

is not the same as feeling. To feel, you must learn to communicate with your body.

In order to allow your body to recover, you must change the way you talk to yourself. Rather than forcing a position, you have to tell your body to let go and give in after a stressful day. This may sound easy, but it is not intuitive. We're so used to working our muscles—no pain, no gain—that simply letting go can be a challenge. With the help of the Miracle Ball Method, over time you will create a new dialogue with your body by giving it different cues. You will ask yourself to feel the weight of the body part resting on the ball and to notice your breathing. By observing these changes, you will help your body break some of those old habits that keep your muscles tight and your stress levels high.

About the Miracle Ball

The Miracle Ball is used differently from any other exercise or physical therapy. When I designed it, I wanted it to be exactly the right size and have the perfect amount of give. It's not magic, but many of my students over the years have called it "miraculous," because it looks so simple. The ball is just a tool to help you feel the weight of different parts of your body. You don't need to push against it, rub against it, or attempt to make it "do" something. The ball is simply there for you to sink into, which will allow your body to heal itself, de-stress, and return to its natural alignment. All you have to do is feel the weight of your body, breathe, and give in to gravity.

These plastic balls are easy to care for and incredibly durable. They are designed for everyone, no matter what body type. They are made from nontoxic PVC and should last for years. Use a damp cloth to wipe off dirt, and if they feel too deflated, you can add air with a standard bike pump.

How to Use This Book

How you use this book will depend on what stage of pregnancy you are in. Here is what I recommend: Begin with Chapter Two, Breathing for Two (or More!). Learning how to breathe properly and understanding the importance of breathing during the ball placements and during your daily activities is integral to finding pain relief, regaining flexibility, energy, and muscle tone.

Next, read about the various ball placements in Chapter Three and the Whole Body Moves in Chapter Four. The ball placements help you relieve tension while the Whole Body Moves help lengthen and tone your muscles.

Regardless of which trimester you are in, you should be able to try most of the ball positions by following the instructions for the variations and finding what works best for your body. (Every pregnancy is different. Consult with your doctor if you have any questions.) You'll notice that one of our models featured in the book does not look pregnant. I made this choice because I wanted to impress upon my readers that starting early—in the first trimester, or even *before* your pregnancy—can help prepare your body for the physical changes of the later months and make it easier to regain your shape postpartum. Start doing the Whole Body Moves and the ball placements before you are pregnant, so that when you do conceive, you will begin your pregnancy with your body properly aligned. (Relaxation can also help with conception.) Plus, if and when certain pain issues do arise, you will already have a routine that you can go to easily and comfortably to find relief.

If you are pregnant now, you should also read Chapter Five about the most common pregnancy complaints. Chances are, you are experiencing at least one—if not all—of them! After each description you will find suggested moves to help you manage the problem. There is also a section on ways to integrate the balls into labor and delivery.

If you've already given birth, you can pick the ball moves and Whole Body Moves that work best for you and combine them with the specific postpartum exercises and adjustments in Chapter Seven. These routines will help you prepare your body to regain its shape and reduce your stress during those hectic early months.

No matter where you are in your pregnancy journey, it's important to follow the instructions carefully for each position—and don't rush. You should also get as comfortable as you can before you get on the balls. Wear loose-fitting clothing and try to eliminate distractions. You can use a yoga mat or blanket if you'd like, but it is not necessary. The method will work in almost any setting, but if you are just starting out, you should try to find a quiet space. This will help you focus on observing your body.

Ideally you would spend 10 to 20 minutes on each ball placement; beginners might start with 5 to 7 minutes and work their way up. However, if you have only a few minutes to spend with the balls, it's better to do just one ball placement carefully and correctly than it is to speed through many. I understand how enticing the promise of relief can be, but moving quickly through the positions will not get you there. If you do the program correctly, the results will come. Remember, this is the easiest "work" you'll ever do. You will actually get more results from working less. You will simply breathe and let your muscles unwind.

Each ball placement and Whole Body Move includes detailed instructions and pictures to guide you. It helps to read the instructions before you begin, and you may even need to refer back to them a few times. This can be very counterintuitive work, so it may not come naturally at first. After you become more attuned to what's happening with your body, there is no need to isolate yourself while doing your ball work. You can get on the ball in the living room with kids running around, or the TV on in the background.

If you experience any kind of discomfort while using the method, take the ball away—pain will trigger your muscles to stiffen even more. Sometimes adjusting the ball slightly—even just an inch—can relieve discomfort and make for a completely different experience. Other times placing the ball under a part of the body that is not experiencing pain can have a more positive effect. If you experience the weight of another part of your body giving in, it can spread relief throughout your body, like a chain reaction. Just play with the different positions to discover which of them works best for you.

Pace Yourself

There are three parts to the method: breathing, ball placements, and Whole Body Moves. You can incorporate different variations of your favorite moves into your regular routine.

Some days you might want to focus on your breathing or Whole Body Moves. Other days, you may just want to work on ball placements. The pacing is the most important thing with this kind of body work. If you apply the body formula to just a few of your favorite ball placements or Whole Body Moves, you will see results. Don't push yourself. If you do less, you're going to get more results.

CHAPTER TWO

Breathing for Two (or More!)

Mindful breathing is one of the best tools to have not just prenatal and postpartum, but for your whole life, and it is an essential component of my method. Breathing is probably the single most important thing you can do for your body to find relief from whatever ails you, whether it's backaches, fatigue, sleeplessness, indigestion, sciatic pain, leg cramps, or poor flexibility. Better breathing burns calories because it improves your metabolism and makes it easier for your muscles to improve the shape of your body. It also makes your skin glow!

As I mentioned in the last chapter, breathing can become challenging with pregnancy because the baby pushes up under the rib cage, squeezing the diaphragm. The diaphragm is not something that most of us think of as being weak or strong. But as the muscle that sits flat across your torso just below your rib cage, it is responsible for pulling air deeper into the lungs—when it's compressed, breathing becomes even more difficult. This means that muscles throughout the body do not receive the oxygen they need in order to remain flexible and unstressed.

There are three components to improving your breathing. Whether you have 5 minutes or 5 seconds, work on your breathing by following these steps:

1. Observe your breath.
2. Make the "S" or "haaa" sound. (See pages 39 and 42.)
3. Note your body's response.

Exhalation is the key to improving your breathing. Any stressors, good or bad (such as the challenges of pregnancy), cause us to hold our breath or take shallow breaths for much of the day, without exhaling fully. When you don't fully empty air from your lungs, you are unable to refill them with fresh air. The more you practice exhaling, the stronger your diaphragm will become, and the more effortless it will be to draw breath over the course of the day.

At first, check in with your breathing throughout the day. You may notice that you don't feel yourself breathing. That is because you are holding your breath or taking shallow breaths. Focus instead on attempting to locate

Good breathing happens naturally if you stop holding your breath.

your breath in different ways. Try lying on your back, and rest one hand on your belly and one hand on your chest. (If you are not comfortable lying on your back, you can do this while lying on your side or propped up on pillows in bed.) Observe your breathing and see if your belly rises before your chest does. Chances are, if you are like most people, you are lifting with your chest first. Your chest muscles are not the most efficient way to bring oxygen to your body. Breathe again, but this time try to start the breath in your abdominal area. Focusing your attention here while resting your hands on your lower belly—this will help you avoid lifting your chest and allow the diaphragm to pull the breath in.

After you learn the following breathing techniques, make one or all of them a part of your everyday life. Spend a few minutes breathing in bed when you wake up, or while waiting at the doctor's office, or in line at the grocery store. It is ideal to do breath work for 15 to 20 minutes per day, but you can start with just 5 minutes. Once you feel comfortable with one or more of these techniques, combine it with the different ball placements and Whole Body Moves.

THE "S" SOUND

• relieves anxiety, muscle tension, and fatigue

Focus on your exhalation in order to improve your breathing. This will strengthen your diaphragm, which is especially important during pregnancy.

1 On an exhale, make the sound of an "S" during the entire exhalation. SSSSSSSSSSSS.

Try to make that "S" sound as loud and as long as you can, but do not force every ounce of breath out of your body.

2 Right before the end of the exhalation, stop and notice any changes in your breathing and start your body dialogue. You may say to yourself: "I feel muscles working that I never felt before" or "I'm starting to breathe more deeply." Take note of the changes and then make the "S" sound again. As you exhale, note if you are using your chest muscles or your jaw and shift the work to your diaphragm. In between "S" sounds, you might feel the breath in your back muscles or in areas that you never noticed before.

3 Repeat the sequence for 5 to 7 minutes, taking time in between breaths to observe your body's reactions. When you feel able to, practice your breathing for 15 or 20 minutes at a time. You can incorporate Seated Body Hang Over (page 153).

Open Mouth Breathing

- **relieves anxiety, muscle tension, fatigue, and TMJ**

Many of us tighten our jaw and strain our upper body when stressed. This breathing technique can release those muscles.

1 To begin, exhale by opening your mouth and making a hushed "haaa" sound as if you were trying to fog up a cold window. Let the jaw give in to gravity. Start your body dialogue: As your jaw loosens, do you feel any other parts of your body release? Resist?

2 When you finish the exhalation, gently close your mouth. (Do not clamp the jaw shut by clenching your teeth.) Just allow your lips to touch and notice if there are any changes in your breathing. Give yourself a few moments to feel your breath.

3 Repeat this sequence for 5 to 7 minutes, taking the time to really observe any changes. I know you are eager to feel improvement, but observation is essential to building a solid foundation. Don't make it difficult—just ask yourself where you are feeling the breath. You may feel some discomfort in your back muscles or feel the need to move or adjust your body. This is because the oxygen is beginning to flow into areas where muscles have been clenched. For an added stretch, incorporate the Head Release for Neck and Shoulders (page 183).

Tapping

Tapping is a technique that brings oxygen to the surface of the muscles, which relieves tension and causes you to breathe more fully. During pregnancy, the weight of the belly combined with your pre-existing alignment issues, can pull the upper body down and forward, rounding the shoulders. This can cause many issues, such as neck and shoulder discomfort and even indigestion. Tapping can work to relax your upper body, making it easier to lengthen your spine, and loosens the muscles that may be preventing your lungs from fully expanding as you breathe. Tapping first thing in the morning is ideal—it allows you a moment of calm before the day gets going. If you can, tap again at night to increase circulation to prevent muscles from stiffening up as you sleep. You and your partner can even tap each other. Just avoid tapping directly on your stomach or on your back or sides at the level of the baby.

1 While sitting, cup your hand and tap your upper chest, above the breast and below your collarbone. (Your fingertips, as well as the sides and bottom of your hand, should make contact with the skin, sort of like a suction cup.) Do this

for 15 seconds. Tap in a circular motion and with the same frequency you would use to applaud. Rather than thinking of pushing down on your body, think of pulling away from the skin. By doing this, you are encouraging blood flow into muscles that are tight.

2 Stop tapping for a moment and notice any changes. Your upper chest may feel warmer or the muscle tension may be lessened. Whatever the sensation, give yourself time to feel

it. Increased awareness of feeling is the best way to improve.

3 Repeat the sequence for 5 to 7 minutes, tapping for 15 seconds and then resting, noticing your body's responses. Then move on to the shoulder, just above the collarbone, and to the side of the rib cage. Repeat the tapping sequence on the other side of your body, this time with your alternate hand.

RELIEVE HYPERVENTILATION

• relieves dizziness, light-headedness

If you begin to feel light-headed, it may mean that you are experiencing a mild form of hyperventilation. This exercise will help you redirect the flow of oxygen to your muscles.

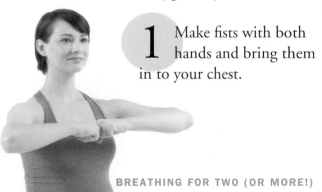

1 Make fists with both hands and bring them in to your chest.

2 Straighten your arms, keeping your fists closed.

3 Repeat the movement several times.

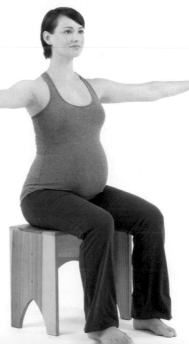

Feeling Light-headed?

As you do your breath work, you may find that your body has a number of different reactions including the desire to stretch or yawn, watery eyes, or dizziness. This is normal, but if you are feeling light-headed, slow down your breath and make sure you fully exhale (it's likely you're inhaling more fully than you are exhaling). If you continue to experience any of these symptoms, you may want to check with your doctor.

CHAPTER THREE

On the Ball

In this chapter, we will cover ball placements under several parts of the body. Choose ball placements that are comfortable. You don't need to put the ball directly under your problem area. Because all of your parts are ultimately connected, there will be a chain reaction no matter what body part you've chosen.

For example, you may be surprised to find that placing the ball under your knee helps your lower back (as long as you're not resisting). You'll have to experiment with different placements to determine which feels best to you.

When you determine which placement works best for you, concentrate on using your *body formula* (weight + breathing = release of tension). While the last chapter was all about breathing, On the Ball deals with the "weight" portion of your body formula. The ball is there to support you so you don't have to "hold" your muscles in a tight position—you can give in to the weight. When you are on the ball your *body dialogue* is important. Most of us have an unconscious dialogue all day that tells us to "work harder" or "push faster." Instead, ask yourself to "give in" or "let go" and feel the weight of your body. If your mind wanders, kindly bring yourself back to the feeling on the ball. Learn to feel the difference between "thinking" about your body and "feeling" your body.

Once you become comfortable with the moves, you can create routines to target specific ailments such as indigestion or back pain. I offer some suggested routines to target common complaints in Chapter Five.

If you are pre- or postpregnancy, or in your first trimester or early in your second, you shouldn't have trouble with any of these ball placements—just stop if something feels uncomfortable. If you have any questions or feel unsure about a position, don't hesitate to consult with your doctor before you begin. Also, for those of you on bed rest, nearly all of these moves will work just fine in bed.

For pregnant women who can't lie on their backs, either because it feels uncomfortable or because they are under doctor's orders not to, there are special variations done in the "PREP" (Pregnancy Required Exercise Placement).

Lying on your back can disrupt the blood flow through the inferior vena cava—the major blood vessel leading into your heart—which can make you feel dizzy or light-headed. If you need to stay directly off your back, simply follow the PREP variations which will show you how to do the moves while the pelvis is slightly raised to one side. This will take the pressure off the inferior vena cava. If you have any discomfort while doing the PREP positions, simply stick to the ball placements that don't require that you be on your back.

Whether you follow a variation or do the basic move, always focus on finding a position where you feel comfortable and where you can breathe naturally. Feeling good is the key to releasing this tension. It's how your body lets you know that things are going in the right direction. Good luck!

Finding Your Hip Joints

- **key area: pelvis**
- **relieves stiff lower back muscles and hip joints**

Before you get on the ball, you need to become more aware of your hip joints. Back and sciatic pain is often caused by tight hip joints, which can pull on your back and cause strain and misalignment. If you don't want to lie on your back, try the PREP variation on page 61.

1 Lie on the floor with your legs outstretched and, without forcing anything, observe how

close your legs, hips, and back are resting to the floor. Don't try to fix anything; just observe and feel.

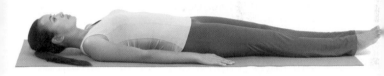

2 Bend your knees and rest your feet on the floor.

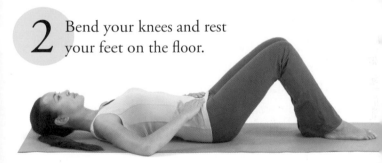

You will probably notice that more of your body now rests easily on the floor. Does your back flatten out? Notice how the movement of your hip joints affects your lower back.

3 Very slowly, repeat extending and bending your knees 3 times. Be aware of your hip joints.

Once you loosen up your hip joints, you will experience relief in your entire back. In addition, when you stand up, you will naturally start to transfer the weight you have been carrying in your back onto your legs, where it belongs.

- **variation to comfortably do ball placements without lying on your back**

Here's a basic description of the PREP, which you can get familiar with before trying the variations listed under each ball placement.

1 Lie down on the floor on your right side, bend your knees, and rest the weight of your body on the floor.

Begin your body dialogue: Notice which parts of your body are resting on the floor and which parts are not. The parts off the floor are ones you are holding tightly. These are the areas that need to give in to help your bones realign. Be aware if you are holding your breath. Make the "S" sound, or use open mouth breathing.

2 When you are ready, take a ball in your left hand, place it on the floor behind your pelvis. Roll back so your left buttock is resting on the ball. Let the weight of your hip rest on the ball. Adjust the ball as needed.

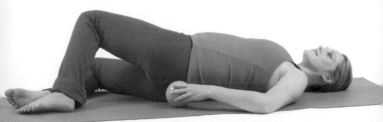

If you feel your back resisting, focus on relaxing your rib cage toward the floor; this will allow your waist and lower back to settle, too.

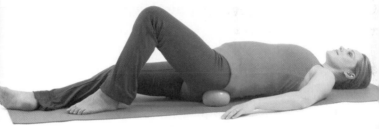

3 Give in to the weight, letting the weight of your hip joint rest on the ball. It's normal to feel your body making slight adjustments. Adjust the ball so it fits snugly under your left hip joint. (Your right hip should be on the ground.) Just

be sure that your pelvis is slanting slightly to the right so there is no pressure on the vena cava.

You'll know that you are doing the movement correctly if you can lie comfortably without feeling like you are struggling to balance or breathe. (If you are having difficulty keeping the ball in place, that means your muscles are tensing.) You can also place the second ball underneath your neck if that feels good to you. After you've completed the move on your left side, switch and try it on your right side. Once you become comfortable with this basic postion, you can move on to the PREP variations thoughout the book.

BACK ON THE BALL

- key area: pelvis
- relieves lower backache; promotes relaxation

Back on the Ball is a great way to relieve lower backaches and gain flexibility in the hip joints and hamstrings. During pregnancy, many women hold their spine in an arch, like a big violin bow. Back on the Ball eases the stiffness in that arch, allowing it to reverse gradually. You don't need to force it; just let gravity do the work. You may feel small adjustments in your body as you rest on the ball. These movements mean your body is trying to find its balance. Listen to your body.

This ball placement calls for just one ball, but if you feel wobbly, unstable, or uncomfortable, please feel free to use two balls for extra support—one on either side of your tailbone. If at any time you feel like you are going to fall off the ball, it means you are holding your breath and have lost the sense of your weight sinking into the ball. If this happens, come down off the ball and then try again.

1 Lie on the floor on your back. Bend your knees and rest the weight of your body on the floor.

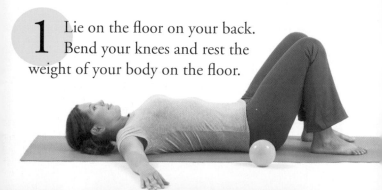

Begin your body dialogue: Notice which parts of your body are resting easily on the floor and which parts are not. The parts that are off the floor are the parts that you are holding tightly. Breathe, making the "S" sound or using open mouth breathing to relax.

2 Take a ball and roll your pelvis to the side. Place the ball in the middle of the back of your pelvis.

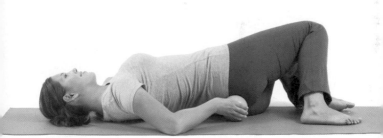

The exact placement of the ball is flexible. You may place it as far down as your tailbone or as far up as the middle of your pelvis. Beginners should avoid placing the ball up to the top of the pelvis, at the waistline—that location is usually the tightest part of the back.

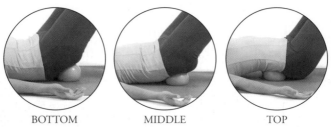

BOTTOM   MIDDLE   TOP

3 Roll your pelvis up onto the ball. Feel the weight of your pelvis give in to the ball.

Notice if the arch of your back feels tight, like a violin bow. If you place the ball under your tailbone, your spine can hang down from your tailbone

HAMMOCK

VIOLIN BOW

tailbone like a hammock, lengthening your back muscles. *Don't fix it; just feel it. Let your body do the work.*

4 Make the "S" sound again to ensure you are not holding your breath.

If you feel that your back is resistant to giving in, focus on relaxing your rib cage against the floor. A stiff rib cage can make it difficult for your waist and lower back to settle. Rest, make the "S" sound, and let your muscles give in.

5 With your pelvis resting on the ball, bring your legs up toward your chest, one at a time, keeping your legs parallel to each other. Give in to the weight of your legs.

If you don't like how this feels, or if your belly is in the way, move your thighs apart. Don't worry about staying perfectly

There are only two responses your body can have to the ball: resisting or giving in.

centered. Give in to gravity for 1 to 2 minutes, if possible. You should feel a gentle stretch in the hip joints and the lower back. Notice if you are holding your breath and make the "S" sound. Feel the weight of your body.

6 With your pelvis anchored on the ball, slowly let your thighs move apart as far as gravity will allow. Do not force them. Rest in this position for up to 2 minutes. This is particularly

useful if you have very tight inner thigh muscles, which can cause knee pain and make it more difficult to stand— especially during pregnancy.

7 With your hands on the outside of your upper thighs, slowly bring your thighs back together. Let your knees follow your thighs, rather than leading with the knees, which is the

tendency. Feel the muscles in the outer thighs gently working. Repeat this movement 3 times. If you can, let your legs to open wider each time.

8 One at a time, return your feet to the floor. Allow your body to rest and breathe, then roll your pelvis over onto your side. Quickly remove the ball.

Extend your legs and let the weight of your body sink to the floor. What do you notice? Did you stop holding your breath? Does your back feel closer to the floor? Do this ball sequence 3 times. This move works well when combined with Seated Body Hang Over (page 153).

1 Get in the PREP position (see page 61).

2 Bend your left knee and let it fall toward your chest. (You can clasp your fingers around the top of your left knee to help it stay in place if needed.)

Release your buttocks muscles and give in to the weight. You'll feel a nice stretch in your lower back. Don't worry about staying perfectly centered. You shouldn't feel like you are struggling to balance. Your pelvis will change position on the ball slightly as your leg comes up. You should feel a gradual stretch around your hip joints and lower back. Once you feel stable, put your foot back on the floor and slide the leg out. Rest and feel the weight of your legs. Repeat the sequence 2 or 3 times. You can move the ball higher and lower along your hip to release different muscles.

3 To get a nice inner thigh stretch, let the left leg fall out to the side as far as you can (for some it may not be that far). Make the "S" sound. Rest in this position and let your inner thigh release. If it feels more comfortable, bend your right knee out to the side.

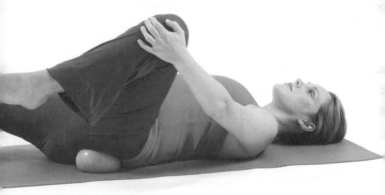

4 With your left hand, slowly bring your leg back up toward your chest. Let your knee follow your thigh rather than leading with the knee so you work the correct muscles. You can also place your hands on the outside of your left buttock to feel the muscles in the outer thighs working. Repeat, letting your left leg slowly fall out to the side 3 times.

5 Bring your left leg down so the foot is resting on the floor. Stretch out your legs and rest. Flex and point your left foot a few times. Notice any changes. Roll over onto your side. Let your body melt into the floor. What do you notice? Did you stop holding your breath? Make a mental note of any changes.

6 Get back into the PREP position (page 61), this time on your left side. Place the ball behind your pelvis and roll back so your right buttock is on the ball. Repeat Back on the Ball with the right leg.

Two Balls Under the Hips

- **key area: pelvis**
- **relieves sciatic pain, knee pain, lower and middle back pain; offers general relaxation and support**

This movement is excellent for sciatic pain. It will give you a great sense of the tightness in your buttock muscles and help you release your hip flexors, which support a considerable amount of extra weight as the baby gets larger. The added strain can make your hip flexors very tight, causing discomfort. This ball placement will give the area a deep stretch.

1 Lie down on the floor and bend your knees, resting both feet on the floor. Take note of your breathing and how your body feels in this position.

2 Rolling from one side to the other, place the balls under each buttock, at the middle of your pelvis (the top being near your beltline, the bottom, where you sit). Make the "S" sound.

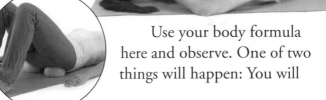

Use your body formula here and observe. One of two things will happen: You will notice nothing (in which case you may be holding your muscles) or you will feel a sense of letting go. Can you rest more easily on the ball? Has your breathing changed? Experiment with moving the ball toward the top of your pelvis and then to the bottom. (See page 68.)

3 Bring your right knee up toward your chest. Let your body rest, resisting the temptation to tense your muscles to stay on the ball.

Then place your foot back on the floor. Do this movement slowly 3 times, then repeat with the left leg.

4 Now bring both knees up toward your chest. Take a few moments to notice any changes in how your body rests on the balls. Are you holding one side of your body more tightly than the other? Try to ease up the side that is clenched, and tune in to your body dialogue.

Can you feel the angle of your pelvis changing in this position? It's okay if you are distracted at times, but continue to develop this deeper dialogue with yourself.

5 With your knees still bent, open up your thighs for a nice stretch, rotating from the hips, not the knees. Feel the weight of your thighs and breathe for as long as it is comfortable. If this movement hurts your knees, you are probably rotating from the

knees instead of the hips. Do not force this position. If it doesn't feel right, skip it.

6 Slowly bring your thighs back together, and let the weight of your legs rest into your body, making sure not to squeeze the knees together. (If your belly is in the way, you can leave your legs a little bit apart.) The legs should return as evenly as possible. Repeat slowly 3 times and breathe.

7 Return your feet to the floor, moving the balls down to your sitz bones, and extend your legs. Feel the legs give in to gravity. You now have the option of going into a hamstring stretch

(Step 8) and quadriceps stretch (Step 9). Or, you can remove the balls one by one and stay on your back to feel the changes in your body.

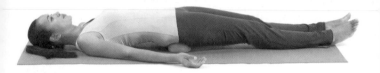

8 Optional: Starting in the position described in Step 6, extend your legs up in the air. Reach with your feet and try not to lock your knees. Keep the weight of your hips on the balls so you feel the give in your leg joints. Bend your knees slightly to feel the weight more heavily on the balls, then straighten them out. Flex and

stretch your ankles.
Slowly let your legs
bend back into your
body. Bring your feet
to the floor.

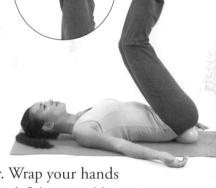

9 Optional: For a quadriceps stretch, remain on the balls and place both feet on the floor. Wrap your hands around the top of your left knee and bring it

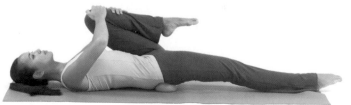

toward your body and extend your right leg. Feel your leg sink into your chest. Return your left foot to the floor, and repeat with alternate knee. To finish, stretch your legs out and remove balls one at a time. Follow with Standing Body Hang Over (page 157).

(page 157)

PREP VARIATION

1 Get into the PREP position (see page 61).

2 Bring your left knee up toward your chest. Feel the weight of your left hip joint on the

ball and then place your left foot back on the floor.
Do this movement 3 times slowly.

3 With your knee bent, open up your left thigh
for a nice stretch, rotating from the hip, not
the knee. If it is more comfortable, you can bend
your right leg to the side. Feel the weight of your
thigh and breathe. If this movement hurts your
knee, you are probably rotating from the knee
instead of the hip. Do not force this position. If it
doesn't feel right to you,
feel free to skip it.

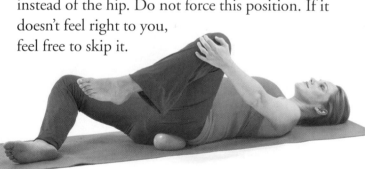

4 You have the option here of adding a hamstring stretch. Try straightening your left leg up in the air while your pelvis rests on the ball. Make sure you are reaching with your foot and that you are not locking your knee. Keep the weight of your hip on the ball so that you feel the give in your hip joint. Bend your knee slightly to feel the weight more heavily on the ball, and then lengthen it up, leading with your foot. Flex and point your foot 2 or 3 times.

5 Place your foot on the floor, slide your leg out, and rest. When you are ready, roll onto your right side and remove the ball. Observe: Do you rest more easily on the floor? Do you feel more parts of your body touching the floor? Has your breathing changed? Repeat the stretch with your right leg. Alternate sides 2 or 3 times.

Ribs on the Ball

- **key area: rib cage**
- **relieves middle back pain, shoulder tension; reshapes waistline**

I call the muscles around the rib cage the "mystery area." Most people don't think of working their rib cage but for many, muscle tension in this area is the culprit behind their back, neck, and shoulder pain. In this move, you should focus on feeling the weight of your rib cage. If you feel straining in your head or neck, rest your head on a small pillow or place the other ball under your neck. Position the ball so that you can let go and breathe. You may need to adjust the ball under your ribs a few times until you find a comfortable position.

1 Begin by lying on your side on the floor. Choose the side that you can roll onto the most comfortably. Bend your knees slightly, but don't curl up into the fetal position. Try to form a nice long line from the top of your head to your hips, not a tight curve.

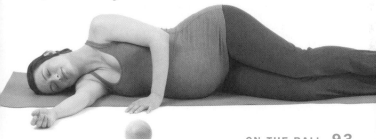

2 Place the ball under your ribs by rolling back slightly, then rolling up onto the ball.

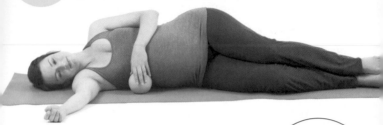

Once you've got the ball in a comfortable position, give in to the weight of your body. If you can, stay on the ball for 2 to 3 minutes, remembering to breathe. As you feel your breathing, you may allow for adjustments.

3 Take the ball away by rolling slightly backward and pull the ball out from the front. Let your rib cage sink into the floor. Is your breathing easier? Do you feel that more of your rib cage is resting on the floor?

4 Repeat going on and off the ball 2 or 3 times on one side, then roll over and try this ball placement on your other side. Notice responses in other parts of your body. In between sides, try the Whole Body Twist (page 172).

KNEE ON THE BALL

- **key area: pelvis**
- **relieves achy knees, tense leg muscles, and sciatic pain; promotes relaxation**

This move is designed to relieve sciatic pain (a very common pregnancy ailment) by adjusting your leg alignment. As you rotate the knee slowly on the ball, you'll ease stiffness in the leg and hip, which takes the pressure off the sciatic nerve and helps realign your hips. The best part: You can do this in bed! (As with any of the ball placements, sometimes simply resting on the ball and feeling the weight can be effective.)

1

Lie on the floor on your back. and place a ball under the back of one knee.

Avoid stiffening your leg. Let your hip joint rotate if that is what it is inclined to do.

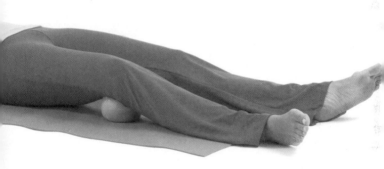

2 Let your thigh muscle give in and let your knee roll outward from the center, keeping it on the ball. Rest on the ball for as long as you feel a release.

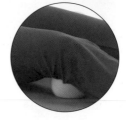

3 Gradually rotate the knee inward until your legs are parallel again.

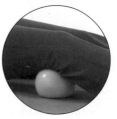

Make the "S" sound and notice any changes. Are your leg muscles easing up at all? Do you feel any reaction in other parts of your body?

4 Very slowly, release the knee to a neutral position and take it off the ball. Rest your leg on the floor and feel any changes.

5 Repeat the move with the other knee.

Adjust the ball to your body, not your body to the ball.

BALL BETWEEN THE KNEES

- key area: pelvis
- relieves hip pain, lower back pain and tension; great to do in bed to relieve stiff legs

This is your go-to exercise for emergency relief of a lower back spasm. Remember your legs have a direct connection with your lower back. Resting the ball between your knees will take the pressure off your legs and ease those tight leg muscles that cause lower back pain. You can do this position in bed, and it may also be helpful during labor.

1 Begin by lying on whatever side is most comfortable. Relax your bottom shoulder and roll slightly back onto your rib cage. Avoid resting too heavily on your bottom shoulder and pulling yourself into the fetal position. Breathe and feel the weight of your body sink into the floor.

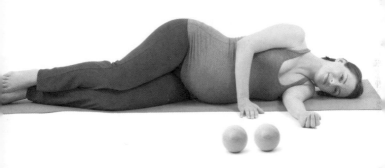

2 Bend your knees at a 90-degree angle. Take a ball and place it between your thighs just above your knees. If it's more comfortable for you, you can put the other ball under the side of your head or neck. Rest in this position and make the "S" sound or do open mouth breathing. Let your top leg sink into the ball; it should feel very heavy and at ease.

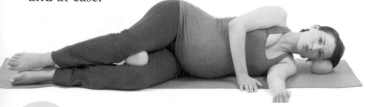

3 Feeling the weight, slide your top knee very slowly a few inches past your bottom knee, allowing the muscles of the inner thigh to rest on the ball. Rest here for as long as you feel comfortable.

4 Slide the top knee back behind, so your knees are even again. Rest here. Repeat this motion as many times as you like, then reverse directions. Take the top thigh and pull it back so that the top knee moves a little behind the bottom knee—just an inch or two.

Focus more on giving in to the weight than on the movement itself. Notice if you start to hold your breath. Make the "S" sound.

5 Lift your top knee just enough to remove the ball. Gradually release the weight of your top leg so it is resting on your bottom leg. Breathe, check in with your body dialogue. Repeat this move 3 times, then roll over and repeat on your other side. This ball placement can bring incredible relief if done very slowly.

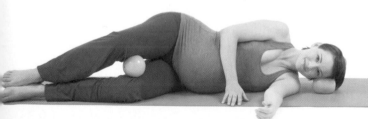

FOOT ON THE BALL

- **key area: pelvis**
- **relieves foot pain, leg cramps, and stiff hip joints; strengthens ankles**

When you are carrying a baby, standing for long periods of time can be tough on your feet and legs. This ball placement targets the feet, easing tension in the muscles throughout the entire leg, which can help with leg cramps. You can also do this ball placement sitting up.

1 Lie on your back on the floor with your legs stretched out. Place a ball under your right knee.

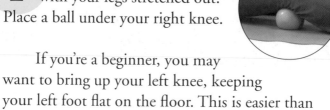

If you're a beginner, you may want to bring up your left knee, keeping your left foot flat on the floor. This is easier than keeping that leg stretched out.

2 Bend your right knee and rest the bottom of your foot on the ball.

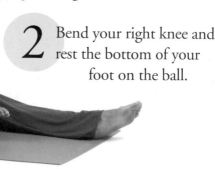

3 Gently move your foot forward and back over the ball for 2 to 3 minutes. Bring your attention to the weight of your foot on the ball.

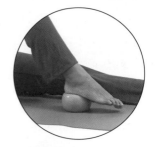

Move very slowly, gradually increasing the distance until you are rolling the ball all the way from your heel to your toes. Remember to let your ankle bend.

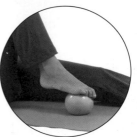

4 Let your leg straighten out, rolling the ball underneath your ankle.

Rest here for a minute or two and notice your breathing.

5 Bend your knee again and repeat this movement 3 times. Feel what happens to other parts of your body. Do you feel the connection to your back? Repeat this same movement with the opposite leg.

1 Get into the PREP position (see page 61).

2 Take the second ball in your left hand and place it under the left knee. Bend your left knee and rest your left foot on the ball. Slowly and gradually move your foot forward and back on the ball.

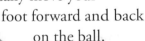

3 Gradually, let your left knee and thigh release outward, letting the left side of your ankle rest on the ball. Rest in this position for as long as you feel comfortable.

4 Gently move your thigh back up, resting the bottom of your foot on the ball again. Roll your foot forward and back over the ball for 2 to 3 minutes.

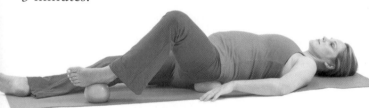

5 Let your leg straighten out, rolling the ball underneath your ankle (or calf). Rest here if it feels good. Give in to the weight of your leg. Breathe.

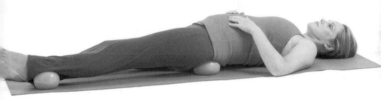

Feel what happens to other parts of your body. Do you feel changes in your back? Repeat the same movements with the right leg.

CALVES ON A STOOL

- **key area: pelvis**
- **relieves lower back pain; strengthens abdominal muscles**

This position works wonders for lower back pain, and can also relieve digestive problems by helping the baby rest comfortably in the pelvic cavity. It is also an ideal exercise for postpartum recovery, since it encourages the abdominal muscles to regain their natural shape, which is important to improving abdominal tone.

You'll need a surface that is about 14 to 16 inches high, such as a stool, bench, ottoman, or coffee table. Your feet should not be higher than your knees and your calves should be roughly parallel to the floor. You want your legs to rest comfortably. The support of the stool takes all the tension off the lower back, which makes breathing easier, because your diaphragm can contract with ease. If you do not wish to lie on your back, do the PREP variation for Calves on a Stool with Legwork (page 121).

1 Lie on your back and rest your calves on the stool, so that your knees and feet are at the same height and your calves are parallel to the floor.

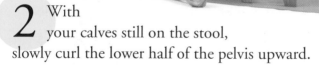

2 With your calves still on the stool, slowly curl the lower half of the pelvis upward.

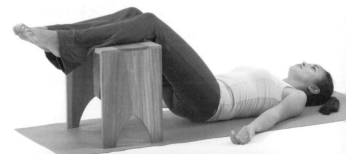

Do not lift your pelvis as though to exercise your abdominals; rather, curl your pelvis as though you are trying to bring your sitz bones up to face the ceiling. Then, use gravity to gradually release the pelvis back down to the floor and feel its weight. Does more of your pelvis rest flat on the floor? This is generally a very stressed area of the body, so take your time with this move. Take note of your breathing and the changes taking place in your body.

3 Do this for 10 to 15 minutes per day to get the best results. Try combining this position with Seated Body Roll Back (page 165).

CALVES ON A STOOL WITH LEGWORK

- key area: pelvis
- relieves leg cramps; aligns hips and legs; reduces stress

This move expands on Calves on a Stool (page 112). It puts your pelvic cavity in alignment with your spine and offers a deeper release of the hip joints, giving your leg muscles a chance to let go of their tension.

1 Lie flat on your back and rest your calves on the stool, so that your knees and feet are at the

same height and your calves are parallel to the floor. Roll your hips to the left, and with your right hand place the ball under your right buttock. Repeat on your left side.

You can always shift the balls around until you find a position that's comfortable for you. I recommend putting them under the fleshiest part of your buttocks—where the hip joint is located. You can always move the balls higher or lower (page 68) but the exact location isn't important. What matters is that the position is comfortable for you and that you are able to feel that the balls are absorbing your weight.

2 Now draw your right knee gently to your chest, clasping your fingers around the knee to bring it in closer. (If your belly is in the way, let your leg move to the side.) Feel the weight on the ball, then let the leg sink back onto the stool. Repeat with the left leg.

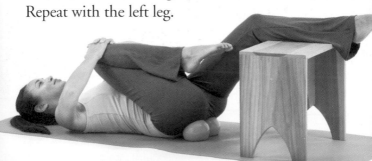

3 With your legs back on the stool, slide both toward you so that your heels are near the edge of the stool. Let your thighs fall open. Allow the weight of your legs to stretch out your whole back and your inner thighs. Rest in this position for as long as you comfortably can.

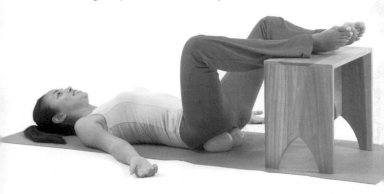

4 Slide your calves back onto the stool, and rolling from side to side, remove the balls one at a time.

Are you resting differently on the floor? Are you breathing differently?

5 To come off of the stool, roll to one side. Rest there for a few minutes. Repeat this sequence 2 or 3 times.

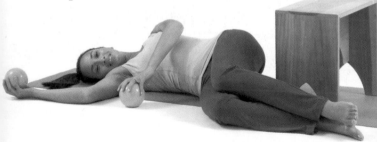

1 Positioning a stool behind your calves, get into the PREP position (see page 61). As you roll back onto the ball, lift your calves onto the stool, making sure your left hip is tilted to one side.

2 Slide your right calf off the side of the stool, gradually letting it lower to the floor,

allowing the right thigh to stretch at the hip. Notice your breathing and the changes in your body.

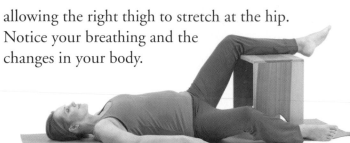

3 Slide your left leg toward you so your heel is near the edge of the stool, and let your left thigh fall open. Allow the weight of your leg to stretch out your whole back and your inner thigh. Rest in this position as long as you comfortably can. Move your leg up to a neutral position. Then drop your leg toward the opposite direction. Rest there and feel the stretch.

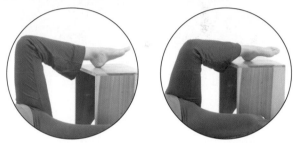

4 Slide your left calf back on the stool. Then roll all the way over to one side taking your legs off the stool. Rest for a few minutes. Repeat the same movements with the other leg.

NECK ON THE BALL

- **key areas: head/neck/shoulders**
- **relieves tension headaches, and neck and shoulder stiffness; promotes stress relief and relaxation**

Neck on the Ball is great for relieving neck and shoulder stiffness and for general relaxation. It also helps improve posture during pregnancy. This is a very versatile move: You can do it lying in bed or lying on your side on the floor. As you feel more confident using the balls, you can combine Neck on the Ball with other ball placements.

1 Lie down on the floor with your legs outstretched.

2 Place one hand under your head and use it to raise your head off the floor. Use the other hand to place the ball under the back of the neck where the base of the skull meets the top of your spine. It is common to "hold" your neck tightly on the ball by pushing your chin down into your neck. Remember to give in to the ball. If the suggested placement for the ball feels uncomfortable, move the ball slightly lower or higher along your neck.

3 Do open mouth breathing to help ease jaw tension, which can also contribute to stress in the neck and shoulders. If you are doing the move correctly, you will notice that you can breathe with more ease. You will also feel an enhanced sense of connection to other parts of your body.

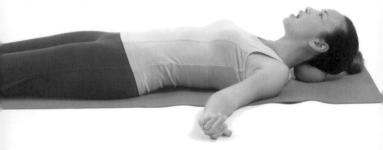

If you feel nothing, chances are you are holding your muscles without even noticing. Also be sure not to press your neck into the ball. Rest on the ball for 2 to 3 minutes if you can, but do not force it.

4 Use one hand to support your head as you quickly remove the ball with the other hand. Ease your head down to the floor slowly. Let your head rest on the floor and take note of your breathing. Did it change? Are you resting any differently on the floor?

5 Repeat this sequence 3 times, spending 2 to 3 minutes on the ball and 1 to 2 minutes off. When you are up on the ball, you can also try turning your neck very slowly from side to side.

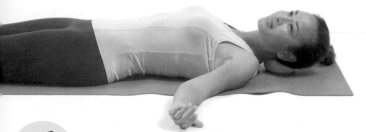

6 When you are done, roll over to one side and sit up using your arms and legs. Notice how your head sits atop your body. Observe any changes. This move works well when followed by Head Release for Neck and Shoulders (page 183).

1 Lie down on the floor on your right side and bend your knees slightly. Your head and rib cage should be resting on the floor as well. Put your right arm out in front of you or wherever it is most comfortable.

2 Place a ball under the side of the head slightly above or to the side of your ear. If this feels uncomfortable, move it

slightly lower or higher. Feel the weight of your head resting on the ball.

3 Do open mouth breathing to help ease jaw tension, which can also contribute to stress in the neck and shoulders.

You may notice that you are breathing with more ease. You will also feel an enhanced sense of connection to other parts of your body. If you feel nothing, chances are you may be holding your muscles without noticing. Rest on the ball for 2 to 3 minutes if you can, but do not force it.

4 Remove the ball and ease your head down to the floor slowly. Let your head rest on the floor and take note of your breathing.

5 Repeat this move 3 times, 2 to 3 minutes on the ball and 1 to 2 minutes off. Repeat the move on the other side.

6 When you've finished, sit either cross-legged on the floor or on a wooden chair or bench. Observe how your head sits atop your body and notice any physical changes.

Shoulders on the Ball

- key areas: head/neck/shoulders
- relieves neck and shoulder tension; eases tension headaches; promotes relaxation

This is a wonderful move to do at the end of the day. Note that placing the balls higher up the back can be more comfortable. The lower down the back you go, the stronger and tighter the muscles are, and thus the more difficult they are to release. So it's often easier to start higher up and work your way down.

1 Lie down on the floor, bend your knees, and rest your feet flat on the floor. Rest your arms on the floor. Notice how you are breathing and which parts of your shoulders and arms are resting on the floor.

2 Take a ball in each hand and place one under each shoulder blade. Do this by rolling onto your right side, reaching over with your right hand, and placing the ball under your left shoulder blade. Then roll up onto that ball, reach your left hand over, and place the ball under the right shoulder blade. Gently roll yourself up or down to move the balls to a place where you can feel your body resting comfortably. Stretch your legs out in front of you and stretch your arms out to your sides, in a "T" position. If you feel any pain in your neck, roll up a towel and place it under your head for support.

3 Rest in this position letting the weight of your shoulders sink into the balls and breathe.

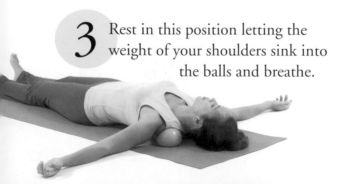

4 Remove the balls one at a time, allowing your body to rest on the floor. Do you notice any changes?

5 Repeat the movements about 3 times. Each time, try to move the balls a little bit lower until you get to the middle of your back. Rest at each spot for 2 to 3 minutes and breathe.

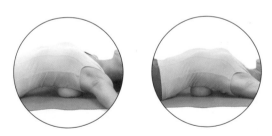

6 If you'd like to continue with this ball placement, put the balls back under the shoulder blades and reach your hands gently up toward the ceiling. Be careful not to tense up. You want to keep the sense of the weight of your body resting on the balls.

7 Then fold your arms across your chest, resting here for about 30 seconds. Exhale deeply and give in to the balls.

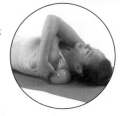

8 Uncross your arms and reach your hands up again toward the ceiling, then back overhead so they are resting on the floor. Rest in this position for another 30 seconds. Finish by bringing your arms to rest at your sides. Breathe.

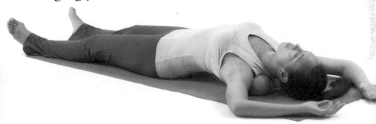

This is also a good time to arch and stretch your back muscles to feel a nice sense of movement and suppleness throughout the whole body.

9 Remove the balls, one at a time. Notice if your breathing is fuller. Spend a few moments here feeling and breathing to deliver oxygen to your muscles. Return to sitting. You can try combining this ball placement with Raising Your Hands (page 162).

1 Get into the PREP postion (see page 61).

2 Place the other ball behind your left shoulder blade with your right hand. With your left arm out to the side, lay your right arm all the way out to make a "T" position (1). Or bring

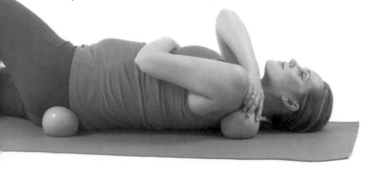

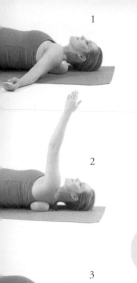

it up toward the ceiling (2) and then rest it alongside your head (3)—anywhere that feels good to you. The ball should roll slightly inward so it's almost in between your shoulder blades. You should feel your rib cage opening up. Breathe in this position for 1 minute.

3 Bring your left arm out to the side. Roll onto your right side and remove the balls. Notice how you feel. Repeat on the other side.

Elbow on the Ball

- **key areas: head/neck/shoulders**
- **relieves stress, tight shoulders, headaches, and stiff neck**

Elbow on the Ball is one of the best ways to loosen the shoulder joints, neck, and lower back all at once. By feeling the weight of your arm as you rest on the ball, your shoulder joint can gently rotate, which loosens the muscles along the upper back. This can ease backaches that may plague you throughout your pregnancy.

1 Lie down on the floor with your arms outstretched.

Notice how your body rests on the floor. If one side seems tighter or more painful than the other, begin with the tighter side.

2 If your left side is tighter, take the ball in your right hand. Make a right angle with your left arm, and then place the ball underneath the left elbow joint.

Let the weight of your elbow—as well as your whole arm and shoulder—give in to the ball. Let your hand rest as close to the floor as your muscles will allow. With practice, your shoulder will rotate enough so that your hand will rest closer to the floor. Rest in this position for 2 to 3 minutes and breathe.

3 Remove the ball. Give in to the weight of your arm on the floor. Is it resting any differently? Compare the arm and shoulder you just worked to your other arm and shoulder. As you give in to the weight of your arm, is it easier to take fuller breaths?

4 Repeat the movement 3 times, 2 to 3 minutes on the ball and 1 to 2 minutes off. Switch sides and repeat with the other elbow.

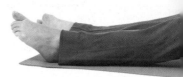

1 Get into the PREP position (see page 61).

2 Take the second ball in your right hand. Make a right angle with your left arm, and then place the ball underneath the left elbow.

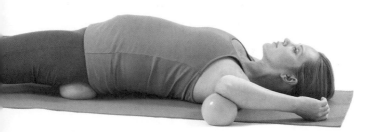

Let the weight of your elbow—as well as your whole arm and shoulder—give in to the ball. Let your hand rest as close to the floor as comes naturally. With practice, your shoulder will rotate enough so that your hand will rest on the floor. Rest for 2 to 3 minutes and notice any changes in other parts of your body. Make the "S" sound.

3 If you find it difficult to keep the ball under your elbow because it keeps rolling out of place, move the ball in toward your body so it rests further up the upper arm an inch or 2.

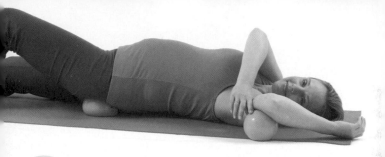

4 Remove the ball. Give in to the weight of your arm on the floor. Is it resting any differently? As you give in to the weight of your arm, is breathing easier?

5 Repeat the movement 3 times, 2 to 3 minutes on the ball and 1 to 2 minutes off. Switch sides and repeat with the other elbow.

CHAPTER FOUR

Whole Body Moves

M any types of exercise mistakenly isolate one part of the body from the rest. We are taught to stretch each group of muscles separately, but our bodies don't work this way. Every movement requires multiple parts of the body to work together as one. Whereas the On the Ball placements help you release tension, the Whole Body Moves help you build strength and tone by moving your body as an integrated whole.

Now that you've been working on the ball and gaining awareness of different parts of your body, it's time to bring in Whole Body Moves. Combining the two will help create longer, leaner muscles that can better adjust to your body's changes throughout pregnancy. They take only a few minutes and you can do them almost anywhere (even while cooking dinner, as I did when I was pregnant). Just one move can help to take the stiffness out of your body and leave you feeling good—no fancy gym equipment required!

Although the Whole Body Moves do not involve balls, the same concepts of breathing and feeling the weight of your body apply. Every time you do one of the Whole Body Moves you may notice a different response in your body, so do them slowly. If you find you are holding your breath, focus on making the "S" sound or the "haaa" sound. Feel the weight of your body. You don't need to "do" much else.

Whole Body Moves are not stretches. I generally avoid using the word "stretch," because I find people push when they stretch, and their muscles shorten, instead of lengthen. As you do the Whole Body Moves, focus on using your weight to pull rather than using your muscles to push.

You might feel muscles stretching that you've never felt before, especially those surrounding the hip joints and those in the back. This is to be expected, so don't be alarmed if it feels awkward. But don't do any move that causes you pain. Instead, make adjustments to the moves, depending on how you feel and where you are in your pregnancy.

Combine one or two Whole Body Moves with your favorite ball placement.

Seated Body Hang Over

- **key area: pelvis**
- **improves breathing and posture; increases flexibility; reduces back pain**

Most people bend over, leading with the upper body. This move is about bending from your root—the pelvis. Rather than stiffening your upper back, hinge at your leg joints. You can combine this move with many of the ball placements in the previous chapter.

1 Sit on a hard chair or bench, feet flat on the floor and slightly wider than hip width apart, hands resting on your thighs.

Ideally your knees should be at the same height as where your sitz bones (the pointy bones at the base of your pelvis) rest on the bench. If you are in your second or third trimester, you will probably need to widen your legs a bit more to make room for your belly.

2 Start by letting the top of your head and neck bend forward, feeling the weight of these parts, then let your torso roll so you are hanging over your thighs, with your arms dangling down to the floor.

Don't let your knees pull in toward each other. This puts tremendous pressure on your feet, ankles, and knees, which can exacerbate sciatic and back pain during pregnancy. Be careful not to arch your back. This will keep you from being able to release your buttock muscles, which is essential to reconfiguring the alignment of your legs. Take note of your breathing. Are you holding your breath? If so, exhale deeply and try making the "S" sound. If you can, rest in this position for about 30 seconds.

3 Slowly sit up, moving from your pelvis. Let your body realign itself, making sure not to hyperextend your back. Connect to your sitz bones. Feel your back muscles lengthening up from your sitz bones. You are creating the muscle tone you will need to carry your baby without unnecessary slouching. Repeat this move 3 times.

STANDING BODY HANG OVER

- **key area: pelvis**
- **relieves tight back muscles and hamstrings; promotes flexibility; reshapes entire body**

This move is designed to stretch and strengthen the whole body. It will relieve hamstring stiffness, lengthen lower back muscles, and flex the hip joints—all of which will help to support the lower back so you can carry the weight of the baby with more ease. You should feel the stretch in your hamstrings, not in your lower back. If your hamstrings are tight, go easy at the start.

1 Stand with your feet a little wider than hip distance apart. Keep your legs straight, but don't lock your knees. This will give you a strong standing base.

Roll your head and body toward your toes, letting your arms hang close to your knees. Start from the top of your head and let its weight lead your torso downward until your arms are hanging close to your knees. Vertebra by vertebra, let your body give in to gravity. Be sure to release your buttocks muscles. This will help you realign your hip joints and lengthen your spine, which will relieve back pain. Focus on trying to bend from the hip joint and roll your pelvis forward over the top of your thigh bones. This is a great place to make the "S" sound to prevent holding your breath.

Your hip joint is here

2 Bend forward from your hips as low as you comfortably can without bending your knees or locking them. Many people avoid straightening their legs for fear of hurting their hamstrings, but constantly bending your knees actually weakens the muscles in your legs and lower back. That said, you should never force any movement.

Be aware of how you feel and hang for only as long as you feel comfortable (a few seconds is fine to start).

3 Roll back up, vertebra by vertebra.

4 Repeat 2 times.

Try to do this move 3 times a day. Eventually you will be able to hang over longer periods as you become more flexible.

Raising Your Hands

- key area: rib cage
- restores energy; improves posture, flexibility, and breathing; reshapes waistline

This Whole Body Move will loosen and lengthen your postural muscles making breathing and digestion easier. It can also prevent low backache and neck and shoulder problems. For best results, do this move as often as possible throughout the day. It will relieve stiffness in your back muscles and keep you from habitually leaning forward.

1

While sitting or standing, raise your hands toward the ceiling without locking your elbows or your shoulders or hyperextending your spine.

You should feel your rib cage lifting up off your diaphragm. You can also tilt your head backward slightly so that you are looking up. This may help you feel the connection with your spine and get more of your body involved. Breathe. It may

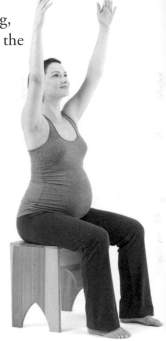

help to look at yourself in a full-length mirror. Are your shoulders up around your ears? Take a breath and drop your shoulders.

2 Bring your arms down gently, without letting yourself fall back into a hunched position.

3 Repeat 3 times or as often as possible throughout the day.

SEATED BODY ROLL BACK

- **key areas: pelvis, rib cage, head/neck/ shoulders**
- **relieves pain in lower back and hip joints, and overall body stiffness**

Depending on your alignment and muscle tone, the weight of your baby tends to draw the whole body downward and push the spine forward, causing the back to arch. This move is designed to reverse that push and relieve tension in the middle and lower back and the neck. It also gives the muscles in the bottom of the pelvis a chance to stretch and strengthen.

1 Sit on a bench or on the floor with your feet together. Roll back gently behind your sitz bones, rounding the front of your body into the back of the body and bending your head forward, so that from the side your body appears to form the letter "C." Allow your leg muscles to release. You should feel this release throughout your body.

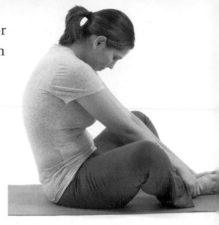

2 Use your pelvic muscles to pull yourself back up onto the top of the sitz bones. Then roll yourself behind your sitz bones once again.

3 Use as much of your body as you can to come back up onto the top of the sitz bones. Make the "S" sound and allow your body to balance in this position for a moment. Notice if you are stiffening any of your muscles. Feel your weight and breathe.

4 Repeat this move 3 to 5 times slowly.

Rib Cage Side Stretch

- **key area: rib cage**
- **reshapes entire body; improves posture and breathing**

The rib cage is connected to nearly half of the spine, so when you lift the rib cage, you are also lifting weight off the lower part of your spine, easing pain and possibly even indigestion. This move will stretch and strengthen the whole spine and tone the muscles of the rib cage, which may help with middle backache. Your neck will lengthen and your breathing will improve. As a bonus, bending your rib cage to the side lengthens your waistline, which gets shorter as your pregnancy progresses.

1 Sit cross-legged on the floor, with your arms hanging at your sides.

2 Keeping both sitz bones on the floor, bend to the right side.

Use your rib cage to guide your head as if you were drawing a big half-circle. Notice your breathing and give in to gravity. Feel the stretch along your ribs and waist. Your arms should hang loosely down the sides of your body; not outstretched, pulling you away from your sitz bones. Don't curl your head and neck forward; you are only arching to the side, so your ear, shoulder, and hip should be aligned.

For a deeper stretch, reach the left arm up and over the right side.

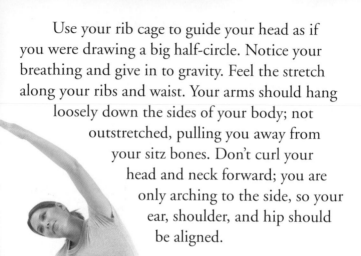

3 Use the rib cage to slowly straighten back up.

You may find that this move lifts the upper back and allows your diaphragm to work more easily. Make the "S" sound, and notice your breathing for a few seconds.

4 Return to sitting up straight with your torso centered over your sitz bones. Do this 2 more times, and then repeat on the left side.

- **key areas: pelvis, rib cage, head/neck/shoulders**
- **slims waist; improves posture; increases energy and breathing; relieves back pain**

This Whole Body Move is a great stretch for pregnant women: It relieves lower back pain, neck and shoulder strain, and opens up the upper chest for easier breathing. All of these benefits will help reduce your stress levels.

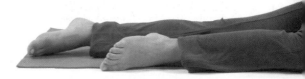

1 Start by lying down on the floor on your side with your knees bent. Slide the top knee in front of the bottom knee and rest the top arm in front of your body. If you feel your head needs support, place a ball or rolled-up towel underneath.

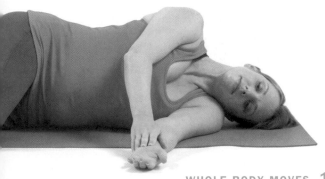

2 Keeping your hips in place, starting with your top hand about an inch off the floor, slowly move your hand over your head and out to the side, dropping it to the floor. Rest here for a few minutes, letting gravity open up your chest muscles and shoulders as you breathe.

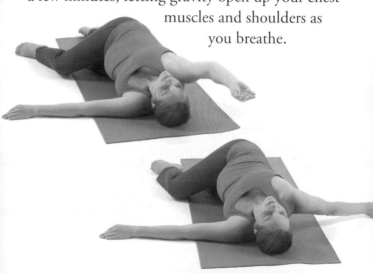

3 Repeat, this time moving your top hand in the opposite direction. Rest and notice any changes. Breathe.

4 To get a nice hamstring stretch, stretch the top leg out in front of you with your foot flexed. Make sure you are breathing and that you are feeling the weight. Repeat rotation 3 times on each side.

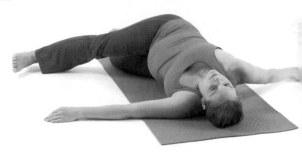

The Posture Pin

- **key area: pelvis**
- **reshapes hips and thighs; realigns entire body; strengthens leg joints, back muscles, and your connection to the pelvic floor (which can improve your sex life)**

The posture pin is a solid cylinder of wood or plastic. It is a great tool for helping you to sit straight atop your sitz bones and find your pelvic floor. Using it is a challenge, but this may be one of the most rewarding positions.

In pregnancy, you tend to get shorter in the lower back and have a rounded posture. A common response is to lift from the upper body, but what you actually need to do is anchor and lift from the lower body. To do this, you need to strengthen your hip joints and your pelvic floor. This move will target these two areas and help lengthen your back, allowing the baby to rest more easily in the pelvic cavity, which not only helps take the pressure off the lower back during pregnancy, but also is the first step to getting your abs back into shape after delivery. A full-length mirror will help you notice if you are forcing your lower back; use it to watch your body's movement and its response to this Whole Body Move.

You can find posture pins on my website (www.elainepetrone.com), but you can also use a standard rolling pin.

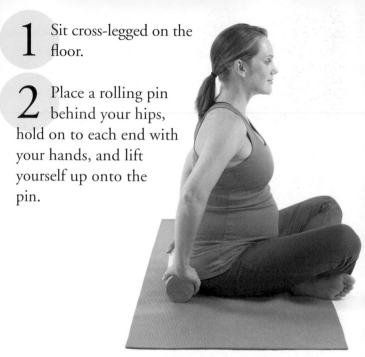

1 Sit cross-legged on the floor.

2 Place a rolling pin behind your hips, hold on to each end with your hands, and lift yourself up onto the pin.

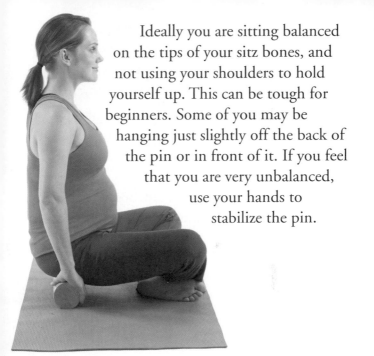

Ideally you are sitting balanced on the tips of your sitz bones, and not using your shoulders to hold yourself up. This can be tough for beginners. Some of you may be hanging just slightly off the back of the pin or in front of it. If you feel that you are very unbalanced, use your hands to stabilize the pin.

Try to *feel* your way to balance, rather than hold what you *think* is good posture. When you are balanced atop your sitz bones, you may notice that your spine is aligned perfectly and your hip joints are getting a gentle stretch. Think again of that stack of children's blocks (page 18). Your neck, rib cage, and pelvis should be stacked similarly.

3 As you balance on your sitz bones, make the "S" sound for 2 minutes, noting any changes in your body.

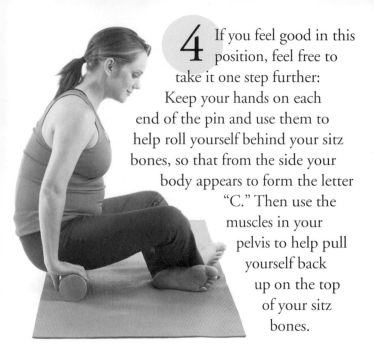

4 If you feel good in this position, feel free to take it one step further: Keep your hands on each end of the pin and use them to help roll yourself behind your sitz bones, so that from the side your body appears to form the letter "C." Then use the muscles in your pelvis to help pull yourself back up on the top of your sitz bones.

5 Repeat this movement slowly several times, remembering to breathe. Make the "S" sound for 2 minutes as you sit and balance.

6 Remove the pin. You should be able to balance atop the sitz bones just as well as with the pin.

Try combining this move with Seated Body Hang Over (page 153).

HEAD RELEASE FOR NECK AND SHOULDERS

- **key areas: head/neck/shoulders**
- **relieves neck and shoulder tension**

This move is designed to loosen tight neck muscles and help your neck and shoulders realign. Plus, it is so simple that you can do it almost anywhere—try it while waiting at the doctor's office or with the TV on.

1 Sit cross-legged on the floor or in a chair.

2 Let your head hang down so your chin is close to your chest. Breathe and give in to gravity.

Rest in this position for a few seconds and notice the relationship of your head to the other key areas of the body—the rib cage and pelvis— that affect your alignment.

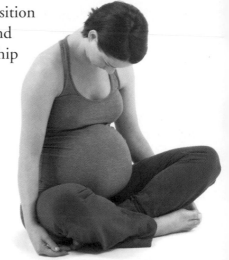

3 Lift your head back up using the muscles in the back of your neck, not your chin and jaw. Neck muscles can get short and contracted from tension, so think about lengthening them as you lift. Notice how you feel throughout your body. Does your head feel aligned? Do you feel taller? Make a full exhalation and feel the lift in your upper chest. Has your breathing changed?

4 Repeat this Whole Body Move slowly 5 to 7 times if you can.

pick-up sticks—you can't control how they land but you can control how you pick them up. This chapter offers you some insight into why these issues arise and provides suggested moves to ease your specific aches and pains.

1. Lower Back Pain: Lower backache is probably the most common pregnancy complaint. The lower back has to support the weight of the baby as the belly pushes forward, so as the baby gets larger, the spine tends to arch and hyperextend. This can cause sciatic pain and even herniated discs. Furthermore, because you get tired from walking around with so much added weight, you will want to sit more, which, unfortunately, increases the pressure on the lower back.

Our hip joints also play a role in lower back pain. The legs connect to the bottom of the pelvis and the spine connects to the top. Tight leg joints cause the pelvis to tip forward, pulling the spine further out of alignment. Thus, an important part of relieving lower backache is reducing the stiffness in the hip joints. Many of the ball placements that address the pelvis can help with lower back pain. Here are three particularly good options:

• *Start your morning off with the Ball Between the Knees (page 100).* Make the "S" sound and rest for 5 minutes on each side. This will relieve leg stiffness.

- *Do the Standing Body Hang Over (page 157).* It is
  ideal for relieving stiffness throughout the entire
  body. It also helps you release your buttocks
  muscles and find your hip joints, which will give
  you extra support in your back when you stand.

- *Or do Back on the Ball (page 65),* which works
  wonders to ease any stiffness in the arch of
  your back and helps your pelvis fall back in
  alignment.

2. Middle Back Pain: As I've discussed,
pregnancy challenges your posture: The increasing
weight of the baby can pull your upper body
forward and down, making it difficult to stay
upright with your rib cage lifted. The result? Sore

muscles in the middle of your back. Also, this downward pull causes the rib cage to rest on the diaphragm, making it more difficult to breathe and bring oxygen to your muscles. Movements that lift the rib cage improve posture and breathing and decrease pain. Here are a few suggestions:

- *Try Tapping (page 45).* Have your partner tap you on your middle and upper back.

- *Do Raising Your Hands (page 162);* it helps lift the rib cage, elongating the neck and back muscles and easing stiffness.

- *Or do Shoulders on the Ball (page 132).* This movement targets tension in the back, shoulders, head, and neck.

3. Neck and Shoulder Pain: It is very common to hold stress in your neck and shoulders, so many women may have pain in these areas even before pregnancy. Stress may cause muscles to tighten, which can result in chronic pain, or—if muscles are extremely tight—pinched nerves. When you are in pain, you tend to hold your breath or breathe with your upper chest instead of with your diaphragm, increasing your tension. Additionally, as your alignment changes, your head and neck are pulled forward, causing more tightness and more stress, and thus, more pain. Here are ways to ease the cycle of neck and shoulder aches:

- *Focus on open mouth breathing (page 42).*
  This will improve the blood flow to the muscles around your rib cage and help you de-stress.

- *Try the Seated Body Hang Over (page 153).*
  The weight of your head will lengthen your neck and shoulder muscles, so don't resist.

- *Elbow on the Ball (page 141)* will rotate the shoulder joint and loosen the muscles surrounding the shoulder.

4. Knee and Foot Pain: Simply standing while pregnant can be a challenge. The added weight of the baby places a great deal of strain on your feet and knees and can affect many other areas.

Any preexisting issues in these areas can also be exacerbated. Here are some great options for addressing pain in your knees and feet:

- *Try Foot on the Ball (page 105)* while sitting. This will ease up the muscles in the ankles and get your circulation going.

- *Two Balls Under the Hips (page 80)*. The pointing and flexing of your foot will help you feel the connection through your knees and hips.

- *Try Knee on the Ball (page 96)* or Foot on the Ball (page 105) to release and oxygenate the muscles in those areas.

5. Sciatic Pain: Most people are not evenly balanced on their legs, so the hips try to compensate, and become tight and shift out of alignment. When the hip joints shift, your bones can actually pinch the nerves on one side of your lower back causing sciatic pain. Here are some moves to give you relief:

• *Do Knee on the Ball (page 96)* while making the "S" sound (page 39). This is a restful position. It also allows the buttocks muscles to loosen and become more supple, which allows your hips to align more evenly.

• *Do the Seated Body Hang Over (page 153).* When you bend forward, notice if your knees roll inward. Try to keep them evenly aligned to ease up the tightness in the hip joint. This Whole Body Move will prevent you from favoring one hip over the other.

- *Or try Two Balls Under the Hips (page 80).* When you are lying on the floor, take time to feel the differences between each side of your body and notice if you are holding your breath.

6. Poor Posture: The hip joints are the foundation of movements for your entire body. When the balance in your body is thrown off by a change in that foundation, everything is pulled out of alignment. This can cause you to develop a rounded posture, or, if you are already predisposed to such a posture, pregnancy can increase the roundness even more. When people feel their posture is suffering, they go to one of two extremes: either they give up and slouch or they hold themselves stiffly upright. Neither action helps. The key is to rebuild the base so you can regain your body's natural alignment. Here are a few solutions:

• *Try the Posture Pin (page 176).* If possible, use a full-length mirror so you can observe how your body balances naturally on the sitz bones. This is a great place to start your readjustment. Remember to make the "S" sound.

- *Do Rib Cage Side Stretch (page 168)* or Ribs on the Ball (page 92). The rib cage makes up half of the spine, so lifting the rib cage also lifts weight off the lower part of your spine, which can help with realignment and good posture.

- *Play with Elbow on the Ball (page 141).* Opening up the shoulders and releasing tension in your upper body is a big part of the posture puzzle.

7. Indigestion: Rounded posture means that your rib cage is hunched forward putting increased pressure on your diaphragm and stomach. This causes a kind of gridlock situation for your digestive system. Unless the diaphragm is free to function normally, you will be plagued with indigestion, which can be exceedingly uncomfortable and makes it difficult to sleep. The key to managing this discomfort is to lengthen the muscles around your rib cage and take the pressure off of the stomach. The following moves can help:

• *Raising Your Hands (page 162)* will lift the rib cage up off the diaphragm so your breathing can flow more freely and your digestion can work more easily.

• *Whole Body Twist (page 172)* will gently improve your posture by lengthening the muscles along your spine, and allow for easier digestion.

- *Do the Rib Cage Side Stretch (page 168)* to lift weight off the lower part of your spine, which in turn will create more room for the diaphragm and ease indigestion.

8. Leg Cramps: Many pregnant women get leg cramps, especially at night, because of the added muscle fatigue and pressure caused by carrying extra weight. If you are prone to cramps, you may be getting into bed at night with stiff muscles and poor breathing. Working with the ball before you go to bed, and focusing on your breathing will ease any tension you are holding in your muscles. When that tension is released, your muscles will loosen, and they will be less likely to cramp.

If you do get a cramp, try not to panic and clench your muscles or lock your knees. Overreacting to the pain will make muscles tighten further, worsening the situation. As soon as you feel the cramp, stop and make a deep "S" sound. This will immediately increase the flow of oxygen to your muscles. And remember to feel the weight of your body even if it is stiffening. Breathe and feel your body relax. Here are a few moves to prevent leg cramps:

- *Choose your favorite ball placement* and breathe mindfully. Make the "S" sound with a deep exhalation. This will immediately increase the flow of oxygen to your muscles.

- *Try Ball Between the Knees (page 100).* Resting your leg on the ball and breathing is a great way to bring feeling to the area and increase the flow of oxygen.

- *Or you can do Calves on a Stool (page 112).* Again, this is about resting your muscles and joints. This ball placement releases tension in your legs, back, and pelvis muscles.

9. Nausea and Morning Sickness:

Unfortunately, there really is no cure for this ailment, but there are ways to make it more tolerable. Breathing is important. Morning sickness is exhausting and breathing will give you more energy. After 5 to 10 minutes of breathing and resting on the ball (maybe even in bed), you may find that you're ready to move around. Include these following suggestions:

- **Practice lifting the rib cage** with Raising Your Hands (page 162). This exercise will improve your posture and your breathing.

- **Calves on a Stool (page 112)** will help to relax your entire body so you can focus on your breathing.

- **Back on the Ball (page 65)** promotes a general sense of well-being.

10. Sleeplessness: If you can't get comfortable, it can be a challenge to get to sleep. The best thing you can do before you fall asleep is to work with the balls and use your breathing to release the tension that has been building in your muscles all day.

Turn off the TV and darken your room. Bring the balls to bed with you and spend some time lying with them in your favorite positions, making the "S" sound or doing open mouth breathing. Just focus on feeling your breath, so your muscles get a chance to relax. Don't try to sleep. Just feel the weight of your body and let your muscles give in. The rest will follow naturally. Here are some suggestions for a good night's sleep:

- **Are you holding your breath?** Make the "S" sound or do open mouth breathing. Observing your breathing is the most important thing you can do to help ease tension so your body can relax.

- **Neck on the Ball (page 124)** is a very versatile move, and it can easily be done in bed. It is great for general relaxation and for relieving neck and shoulder stiffness.

- **Try Ball Between the Knees (page 100)** lying on your side to release the leg muscles. Afterward, you may want to place a pillow between your knees for extra comfort while sleeping.

11. Fatigue: If you are having difficulty sleeping at night, you are going to feel fatigued during the day. However, poor breathing and excess muscle tension can also contribute to general tiredness. Holding your breath is hard work. And when you hold your breath, your muscles don't receive the oxygen they need to function properly. When certain muscles don't work properly, others have to take over, and they eventually become overworked. Overworked muscles are tight and tense, and muscles that are tense get tired faster.

Fatigue can make it difficult to get things done, which can in turn lead to feeling anxious and overwhelmed. Anxiousness sparks the cycle of pain in your body, which causes more tension, and thus, more fatigue. To stop the cycle of pain, you need to focus on breathing and easing your muscle tension. Try these moves when you feel like your energy levels are low:

- *Make the "S" sound.* Don't worry about the volume of the sound. Just do whatever feels comfortable. Rest in your favorite ball placement and breathe.

- *Try Seated or Standing Body Hang Over (pages 153 and 157).* Both of these moves relieve stiffness throughout the entire body. Plus, they are convenient, do-anywhere moves that provide a quick fix.

• *Calves on a Stool (page 112).* Elevating your legs will ease tension in the muscles, but the most important thing is to notice your breathing.

12. Headaches: What do you do when you feel a headache coming on and you can't just pop a pill? You need to start listening to your body. If you listen, you will realize that it's giving you warning signs, and recognizing those signs can prevent a headache from coming on.

Most people react to feeling a twinge of pain by tensing up and holding their breath (or breathe with only their upper chest). Notice if this is happening and use your body dialogue.

Tell yourself to soften your jaw (exhale gently). Oxygen will begin to flow to blood vessels and your jaw tension will loosen. Jaw clenching is a common cause of headache and TMJ. Start by taking note of your body.

As you become more observant and work to change your body's natural response patterns, over time your body will do these things naturally and you can avoid pain. This is the perfect example of the importance of the body dialogue. Headaches are very specific to the individual, so you can choose any ball placement as long as you breathe and observe your body. Here are three ways to start:

- *Try open mouth breathing and Tapping (pages 42 and 45).* Be aware of any muscles you are tensing up. This is something you can do almost anywhere.

- *Do Neck on the Ball (page 124)* if it is comfortable for you. Easing neck muscles can promote relaxation.

- *Try Ball Between the Knees (page 100).* In addition to feeling and breathing, placing a ball between your legs may alleviate some of the pain in your head by helping you relax your entire body.

13. TMJ Syndrome: Referring to the two joints connecting your jaw to your skull, TMJ can be any pain in your jaw muscles. Jaw muscles are extremely strong—and they can hold a lot of tension. A common reaction to stress or pain is to tighten the jaw. A stiff jaw fuels even more stress throughout the body, causing tightness and discomfort to spread—often to your back and neck.

First notice if you are clenching your jaw. Once you feel it, you can fix it. If you are clenching, open your mouth and exhale. Do this often throughout the day. These moves can also help:

- **Neck on the Ball (page 124):** Breathing in this position will help you focus on feeling the weight of your jaw. Combine with open mouth breathing.

- *Try lying on your side* and placing a ball under your head, near your temple. Combine with open mouth breathing and feel the weight of your jaw.

14. Uterine Cramps: As your baby grows inside you, your uterus stretches and expands, often causing cramps. After delivery, your uterus, which is a muscle, contracts vigorously in an attempt to regain its original shape. This is natural, but it can be very intense. Try these moves to find relief:

- *Ball Between the Knees (page 100)* promotes all-over relaxation, which will offset stress you are feeling from the discomfort of the contractions.

- *Neck on the Ball (page 124)* is great to do in bed. It will help you de-stress and focus on breathing through the pain of the contractions.

- *Calves on a Stool (page 112)* will encourage your internal organs to rest back in the pelvic bowl. It will help your abdominals to flatten as well.

Carrying Multiples

When you're pregnant with multiples, everything doubles (or triples!)—your size, the strain on your lower back, your curved posture, difficulty breathing, your hormonal swings, morning sickness, indigestion, sleeplessness.

Your shape changes drastically because your abdominal muscles have to stretch so much more. Your labor is much more of a challenge and of course your doctor is on alert for early delivery. That's why it is essential to start working with the ball earlier to prepare for what's ahead and to help offset the more extreme changes in your body's balance and alignment. Don't wait until your mobility is compromised (as you grow larger, you may need to do a lot of your ball work in bed and your breath work lying down). Focus your attention on these positions:

- *Do Two Balls Under the Hips with Quadriceps Stretch (page 80)* to activate your hip joints, and then combine it with Seated Body Hang Over (page 153).

- *As you get larger,* lie on your side and try Neck on the Ball (page 124).

- *Ball Between the Knees (page 100)* is great for leg cramps. If you're on bed rest (or just tired) this works great in bed.

- *Foot on the Ball (page 105)* will help offset the tension caused by walking around with all that extra weight.

- *Use breastfeeding (page 229)* as a time to breathe and rest.

Labor and Delivery

Everything you've been learning in this book has been preparing you for labor. One of the messages of this book is that you can't fight your body. If you resist, your pain will persist. Whether your contractions are 20 minutes apart, or 20 seconds apart, use the time in between to become aware of any parts of your body that you are clenching or overworking. Use your "S" sound during or between contractions.

To have a successful labor, you need a combination of strong breathing and functional, supple muscles. Remember: Any tension from fear worsens tension in your muscles, making it difficult to breathe and causing more discomfort. Be aware of your thoughts and focus on staying relaxed. Your body knows what to do—just surrender.

The balls can be a great tool for finding relief and relaxation during labor. Take the balls to the hospital with you and use them between contractions.

Throughout your labor, check in with yourself and focus on your body dialogue. Such mindfulness can help you cope with the experience. If you can, do a ball placement. For example, to keep yourself calm, you can place the ball between your thighs and practice making your "S" sound. Let the top leg rest on the ball and allow your muscles to ease up. It will help conserve your energy for when it is time to push.

Here are some suggested ball placements to use during labor or in between contractions:

- **Do Ball Between the Knees (page 100)** or move the ball up slightly so that it rests between your thighs. This will ease pressure on your pelvis and legs.

- **Do Neck on the Ball (page 124).** You can also try this on your side.

- **Focus on your breathing.** Make the "S" sound and pay extra attention to your exhalations.

- **Do Shoulders on the Ball (page 132).** This will open up your chest to allow your breathing to flow more smoothly.

If you are having a caesarean, many of the same rules apply. Use your breathing as best as you can to help your body relax before the surgery. Place a ball between your legs and make a long "S" sound. This will keep you calm and help your body relax.

After delivery, to help myself relax, I did Calves on a Stool (page 112) using the tray table by my bed as a bench. You can even bring the balls to bed with you to help you get to sleep.

Because the Miracle Ball Method is not traditional exercise, most physicians will allow you to do ball work fairly quickly after delivery, including a caesarean.

CHAPTER SIX

Reshaping Your Body After Birth

Having a baby is a life-changing experience filled with joy, but there is also a lot of stress. Plus you may still be experiencing pain from delivery and feeling the additional pressure to do it all: to reshape your body, care for your baby, and possibly rekindle your relationship with your partner. It's easy to become overwhelmed and feel that your time, and in many ways your body, is no longer your own. Although your baby is now your biggest priority, it is also critical to find a few minutes to focus on yourself. Relieve stress, ease aches, regain confidence in your body—you have all the tools you need right here in this book.

My doctor said I recovered faster from my pregnancy than most, especially after having twins, and I know I have the Miracle Ball Method to thank. Simply lying down and breathing may not seem like it would have much of an effect on your figure, but it really is the first step to remaking your body. As you use the balls to adjust your alignment, you are creating a new infrastructure that will form the basis for your body's shape. If you can realign your skeleton and increase the supply of oxygen to your muscles, you will not only reduce muscle pain, but you can also prepare to start exercising again.

Just as with pregnancy, there are many physical issues that can arise during the postpartum period. In this chapter, we'll cover breastfeeding and reshaping your body. But you should feel free to revisit any of your favorite ball placements to achieve overall relaxation and tension relief. And if you are still suffering from things like fatigue (from lack of sleep) or back pain (from carrying your new baby around all day), refer to my recommendations for these conditions in Chapter Five.

Getting Your Body Back

Many women come to me feeling frustrated after giving birth. They are working hard at the gym. They are crunching and crunching, hoping to flatten their bellies, but they are not seeing results. It is very common to get discouraged because exercise doesn't seem to be working. Pregnancy can cause you to lose track of certain muscles without even knowing it. By stimulating feeling in the body again, it becomes easier to integrate those forgotten muscles into movement. Once you learn to feel your body, you can improve it. I saw a famous coach speaking on television who said, "I don't train the muscles. I train the nervous system." That is the trick—muscles will only do what the brain tells them to do.

After carrying and delivering a baby, certain muscles are overworked, making them larger and tighter, while others are underworked. This imbalance can last beyond your pregnancy, and affect your muscle tone and overall shape. As discussed, if muscles are tight and stiff they shorten and are resistant to the adjustments that need to take place in order to change.

You need to relieve the excess tension in your muscles so you can release your bones to realign themselves. *The Miracle Ball Method for Pregnancy* has explored areas of the body that get out of alignment during pregnancy. Now it's time to focus on realigning your body without the extra weight of a baby. You need to help your body engage the muscles that have been affected by pregnancy—most notably your abdominals—if you want them to improve.

The best way to regain your shape is to get (back) on the ball. Reducing tension in the muscles may seem counterproductive, but it is not. You need to regain your alignment before your muscles can fit properly onto your skeletal infrastructure. Proper alignment allows the tension in the body—especially in the back—to release. When those muscles release, they lengthen, which, in concert with tipping the pelvis back into position, creates space for the abdominal muscles to flatten back into the body. You can crunch and crunch all you want, and your muscles will get stronger, but without realignment, the abdominals will continue to protrude, and your belly will never get flat.

As you begin the process of realigning your body, focus first on relaxing and realigning the pelvis. This will allow all the internal organs to rest in the pelvic bowl to help you recover from the inside out. Along with the postpartum exercises outlined in Chapter Seven, you can do any of the ball placements that address the pelvis.

I especially recommend Two Balls Under the Hips (page 80) and Calves on a Stool (page 112).

Two Balls Under the Hips (page 80) is also good for rebuilding the connection between your hips and legs, as is Finding Your Hip Joints (page 58). As you reconnect with your pelvis and hip joints, you will attain a more solid foundation for movement. As your legs begin to anchor you better, you will be able to lift up the other key areas of the body—the rib cage and the head and neck—and your breathing will improve.

As always, your breath will act as the fuel to help you regain your energy. Ball placements and Whole Body Moves lift your rib cage and release shoulder and neck tension, which will lead to easier breathing. I particularly recommend Ribs on the Ball (page 92) and Shoulders on the Ball (page 132), as well as Raising Your Hands (page 162). As you do these moves and ball placements, notice if you are holding your breath. Make the "S" sound or do open mouth breathing. It is possibile to burn calories and reshape your muscles with breath work alone.

Breastfeeding

Though breastfeeding your baby can be a wonderful bonding experience, it can also be frustrating and stressful—especially during the first few weeks. I was like many first-time moms— at first breastfeeding didn't work out. I was tired and I just wanted to give a bottle to someone else and go to bed. But eventually, I found it was actually easier on me and the babies were happier. After I got the hang of it, I found it to be a relaxing time, and often the babies and I would fall asleep together. You have to decide what works best for you, but any time you spend feeding can be used to breathe and rest on the ball. This can even be done in bed. Here are three ball positions to try:

1. Place a ball between your shoulder blades as you sit back with your baby in your arms. Remember to pay attention to your breathing.

2. Lie on your side and place a ball between your thighs when you bring your baby into bed with you. Let your legs relax into the ball and make the "S" sound.

3. Whether lying or sitting, you may like the feeling of having a ball behind your neck for support. Relax along with your baby and and do open mouth breathing.

Making Time for the Method

Even if you have only 5 minutes, you can do a little ball work; you can do Whole Body Moves any time you have a spare moment. If you have other children at home you can lie on the floor while they play and do many of these ball placements.

If you have only a short time to spend on the balls, use it to reconnect with your head, rib cage, and pelvis and to focus on your breathing. For example, you can do breath work, along with Seated Body Hang Over (page 153), while sitting at your kitchen table. Or you might use the ball when you wake up in the morning. Place it under your neck and do open mouth breathing to relieve neck and shoulder tension and TMJ pains, and reduce stress. It will also invigorate you for the day ahead.

If you have 10 minutes to spare, spend a little more time in each position, placing the balls

The most important element of this method is learning how each part affects the way your whole body looks and feels. Make a point of letting all your body parts move. Dance. Be creative. Play.

under one of your favorite key areas. Your body will feel different after delivery, so take time to notice what you feel. If you are extremely tired, use your time on the ball to rest and let your body's weight do the work for you. Sometimes we are so agitated we don't know how to rest, which is only more aggravating. Remember: You don't have to feel relaxed to relax. If you are stressed and feel like the method will not work, just give it a try.

Simply resting your neck on the ball is so easy to do but don't rush it—enjoy it. Get on the ball and allow the muscles of the neck to ease up. When you go back to sitting or standing again, notice if you are balancing differently over your legs.

Even if you have 15 or 20 minutes or more, you may want to use the whole time on one ball placement, which can be very beneficial. For instance, you could only do Back on the Ball (page 65) to fully reconnect with your pelvic muscles. Another option is to work with the ball for part of the time, and then move on to the postpartum exercises in the following chapter. This combination will enable you to tone and gain flexibility in your muscles at the same time.

CHAPTER SEVEN

Postpartum Exercises

The *Miracle Ball Method for Pregnancy* has been preparing you to reshape your body after birth. Continue doing the moves you enjoy. Maintain your breathing (remember, breathing properly actually burns calories!) and keep working on aligning your body. Once you have recovered from your delivery, add the following exercises to your routine. They are designed to expand on the ball work, and they will specifically target your abdominals. I developed these postpartum exercises as a routine, beginning with a warm-up that can flow directly into the ball placements. You can do the whole sequence or simply pick the elements that feel the best.

Keep doing the ball work and Whole Body Moves you enjoyed during pregnancy. They will make these positions more effective.

- **key areas: pelvis, abdominal muscles**
- **brings awareness to the abdominal muscles**

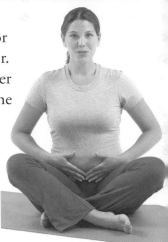

1 Sit on a wooden chair or cross-legged on the floor. Rest your hands on your lower belly between your pubic bone and navel. Become aware of the muscles under your hands.

2 Begin to make an extended "S" sound,

using these muscles to squeeze your entire breath out.

3 Feel your belly fill up with air. Feel your responses and then repeat. Do this for 3 to 5 minutes.

4 In between "S" sounds, let your head bend forward, feeling the weight of your head and neck. Using the muscles at the back of the neck, raise your head up slowly. Repeat that 3 to 5 times, feeling the connection down to your sitz bones.

BALL UNDER KNEE

- **key areas: leg joints, back muscles**
- **relieves knee pain; lengthens waist**

1 Sit cross-legged on the floor. Extend one leg out in front of you and place the ball under that knee and rest your hands on top of your thigh. Feel the weight of your leg and let the muscles ease up.

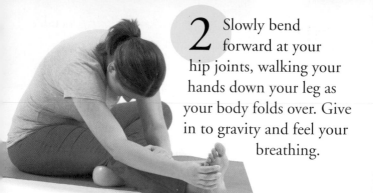

2 Slowly bend forward at your hip joints, walking your hands down your leg as your body folds over. Give in to gravity and feel your breathing.

3 If you are too tight to extend over your leg, just hang your head and walk your hands down as far as they will go comfortably. Gravity and your breath will allow muscles to become more supple.

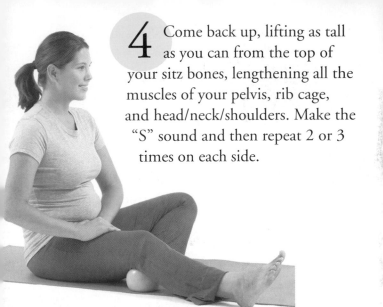

4 Come back up, lifting as tall as you can from the top of your sitz bones, lengthening all the muscles of your pelvis, rib cage, and head/neck/shoulders. Make the "S" sound and then repeat 2 or 3 times on each side.

V-SIT

- **key areas: lower abdominals, pelvis**
- **strengthens pelvic floor, supports lower back; lengthens thighs**

1 Sit on the floor with your legs extended in a wide V and your heels on a line. If you have a wood floor, use a line from one of the boards as a guide. Otherwise it can be helpful to place a piece of tape on the floor.

2 Activate your abdominals by making the "S" sound. If

you want, place your hands above your pubic bone. Feel the muscles contract toward your lower back.

3 Roll back as far as you can, keeping your heels on the line. When your feet begin to move, return to sitting atop your sitz bones by squeezing the muscles at the bottom of your pelvis around your sitz bones. Repeat sequence 2 or 3 times. This move will lengthen the muscles throughout your entire body.

EXTENDED BODY ROLLBACK

- key areas: pelvis, rib cage, head/neck/shoulders
- relieves lower back pain, tones back muscles, improves posture

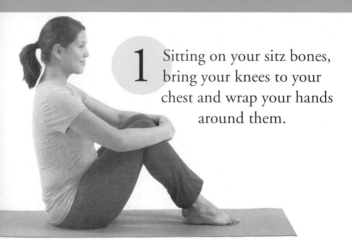

1 Sitting on your sitz bones, bring your knees to your chest and wrap your hands around them.

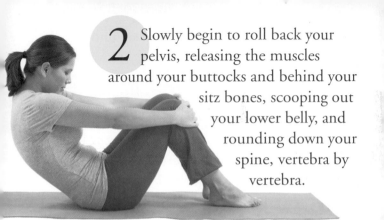

2 Slowly begin to roll back your pelvis, releasing the muscles around your buttocks and behind your sitz bones, scooping out your lower belly, and rounding down your spine, vertebra by vertebra.

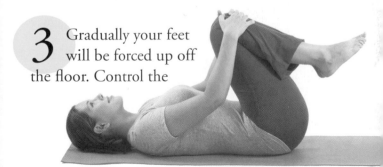

3 Gradually your feet will be forced up off the floor. Control the movement with your back muscles, rolling down gently and slowly until your head touches the floor.

4 Bring yourself back up using your pelvis muscles and abdominals, pressing your back into the floor. Allow your knees to press against your hands. Come back up to the tips of your sitz bones. Repeat the sequence 3 to 5 times. Eventually you can use momentum to roll yourself back up.

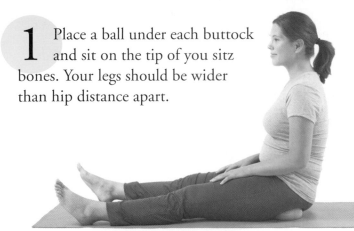

1 Place a ball under each buttock and sit on the tip of you sitz bones. Your legs should be wider than hip distance apart.

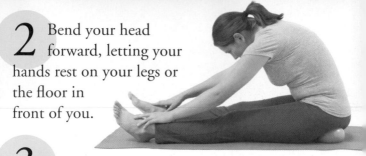

2 Bend your head forward, letting your hands rest on your legs or the floor in front of you.

3 Hinging at your pelvis, stretch your hands toward your feet over your thighs. Reach as far as you can and rest there. Remember to breathe.

4 Use your pelvic muscles to curl up and come all the way back up to sitting, beginning with your pelvis, then your rib cage, with your head and neck coming up last.

Hip Dancing

- key area: pelvis
- gain flexibility through back and legs, tones abdominals

1 Place two balls under your sitz bones. With both feet on the ground, lean back on your elbows.

2 Tip your pelvis forward and back 3 times, feeling the "wheels" of your pelvis turn.

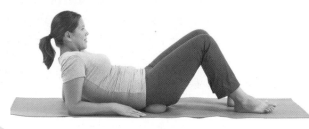

3 Then move your hips side to side 3 times. Repeat the sequence 10 times.

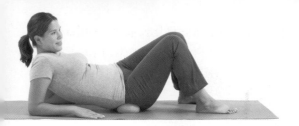

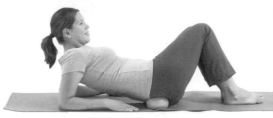

4 Lie down on the floor and remove the balls one by one. Breathe and feel the release in your hips. (You can also incorporate Two Balls Under the Hips, page 80.)

Hamstring Stretch

- **key areas: pelvis, hamstrings**
- **increases flexibility and strength in leg muscles, lengthens lower back muscles**

1 Sit on the floor with your knees apart and place a ball under each buttock, right where your buttock connects to your hamstrings.

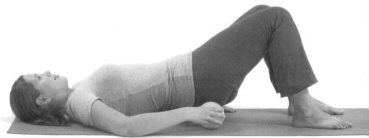

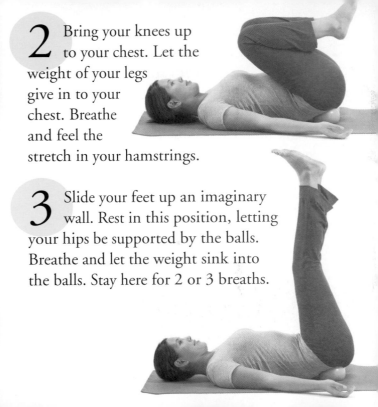

2 Bring your knees up to your chest. Let the weight of your legs give in to your chest. Breathe and feel the stretch in your hamstrings.

3 Slide your feet up an imaginary wall. Rest in this position, letting your hips be supported by the balls. Breathe and let the weight sink into the balls. Stay here for 2 or 3 breaths.

4 Turn out your right leg and place the side of your right ankle on top of your left thigh, holding your left thigh with your hands. Gently pull your left knee to your chest. Rest. Unbend your leg and return your feet to the floor. Rest your weight on the balls. Repeat with your left leg.

5 Place both feet on the floor and slide out both legs. Stretch your hands up toward the ceiling and rest them on the floor over your head. Alternate stretching your left foot and your right hand, lengthening your waist, hips, and thighs. Feel the changes in your body. Switch sides and repeat.

Whole Body Twist with Ball Under the Rib Cage

- **key areas: rib cage; shoulders**
- **improves posture; facilitates breathing; loosens rib cage**

1 Begin by lying on your left side on the floor with your knees bent. Slide your top knee in front of your bottom knee. With your right hand, place a ball in the middle of your upper back.

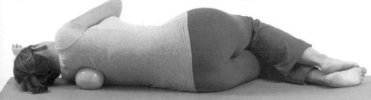

2 Keeping your hips centered, roll up onto the ball, letting your top arm fall back with you gradually. You should feel the weight of the arm as the shoulder begins to stretch. Don't hyperextend your spine.

3 Lift your right arm an inch above the floor and move it slowly in an arc over your head.

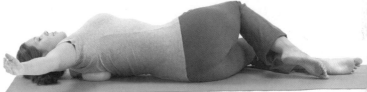

Remember, you will get much more out of the stretch by going slowly and breathing fully.

4 Roll over and repeat the exercise on your other side. The ball may move further up your back. As long as you are still feeling a release, there is no need to adjust.

5 Alternate sides 2 or 3 times.

A Method for Life

After doing these postpartum moves, you may feel ready to start exercising. As you begin, be aware of what you have learned from the Miracle Ball Method. For example, when working out, notice if you are holding your breath or stiffening up certain parts of your body. You can use the balls after your workout to release any tension that has built up.

You can also integrate parts of the Miracle Ball Method into your everyday life, well after your postpartum recovery. For example, during a stressful moment, take time to focus on your breathing. Or, loosen up your muscles by doing a quick Standing Body Hang Over (page 157)—maybe while cooking dinner or playing with your kids. You can use the balls to recover from a busy day at work or to release tension from chasing after your children. You can use the method when you need a moment of restful time alone, with your partner at the end of the day, or while spending time with your children.

Your body knows how to recover from whatever ails it. This book teaches you to listen to your body and allow it to make the adjustments it needs. The Miracle Ball Method of breathing and movement will carry you forward into the rest of your life, any time you need to reduce stress, relieve pain, or reshape your body.

Index

(Page references in **boldface** refer to step-by-step instructions for positions and moves.)

Acknowledgments

Thanks to my students who help me understand how the body improves, moves, and heals. Thanks also go to my children, John, Lucas, and Rose. Although they have given me years of joy, there has also been stress. They used to laugh at me but now that they are grown-up with some stress of their own, we all make the "S" sound together.

If it weren't for the amazing people at Workman Publishing—Peter Workman, Suzie Bolotin, Cassie Murdoch, Maisie Tivnan, Janet Vicario, Yin Wong, Jen Browning, Barbara Peragine, Julie Primavera, Page Edmunds, Anne Kerman, Carol White—my vision would still be locked within the four walls of my classroom. Thanks also to Elizabeth Miersch for her editorial guidance.

And of course, thanks to my friend Jane who introduced me to my agent, Bob Silverstein. From that moment, the ball was rolling. (No pun intended.)